HELKAT LEGACY CO. ✦ BORN OF STORMS

BEHIND THE PATCH THE STORM NEVER STOPPED RIDING

Helen "HelKat" Parkins

—— HELKAT LEGACY CO. ——

BEHIND THE PATCH

One Woman's Outlaw Road To Freedom
By HelKat, All rights reserved.

BEHIND THE PATCH
©2025 Helen "Helkat" Parkins
All rights reserved.

No part of this publication may be reproduced, stored in a retrieval system, or transmitted in any form or by any means, electronic, mechanical, photocopying, recording, or otherwise, without prior written permission of the publisher, except for brief quotations used in reviews or scholarly works.
Brief quotations are encouraged for the purposes of education and review.

This book is intended for educational and informational purposes only and does not constitute legal, medical, or psychological advice. The reader should consult a licensed attorney, licensed counselor, or other qualified professional for advice specific to their situation. The author and publisher accept no liability for actions taken or not taken based on the contents of this book.

This book is available in multiple formats and editions.
Cover and interior design by Helen "HelKat" Parkins.
Published by HelKat Reflections LLC and HelKat Legacy Co

www.helkatreflections.com
Email: bikerbosscoaching@gmail.com

Printed in the United States of America
First Edition
ISBN: 979-8-218-91532-2

──── HELKAT LEGACY CO. ────

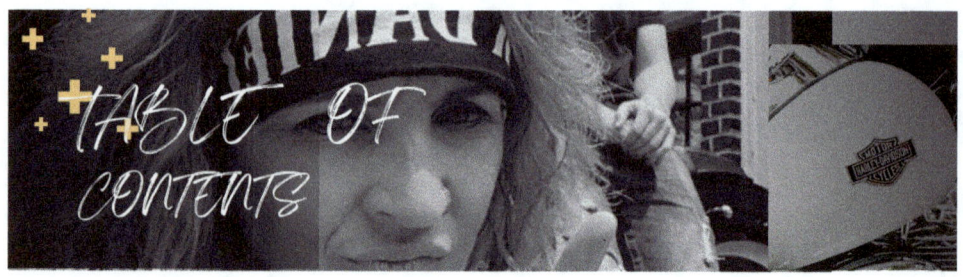

TABLE OF CONTENTS

PART I — BORN INTO THE ROAR

1. Born into the Roar 11
2. The Patch, The Myth & The Woman......................... 23
3. Storm-Born Survival 37
4. Prospecting Ain't for the Weak 53
5. Raised by the Wind 59

PART II — LOVE, LOYALTY & LOSS

6. The Weight of an Ol' Lady 72
7. Heartstrings, Heartaches & Devotion 87
8. Sacred Smoke 98
9. Knives Behind the Patch 107
10. Family by Fire 116

PART III — CHROME, CHAOS & RECKONINGS

11. Chrome & Shadows 126
12. War Stories & Wounds 134
13. Storm Born — Illness, Identity, and
    the Cost of Strength 144
14. Women Who Ride; Faith in the Rearview 157

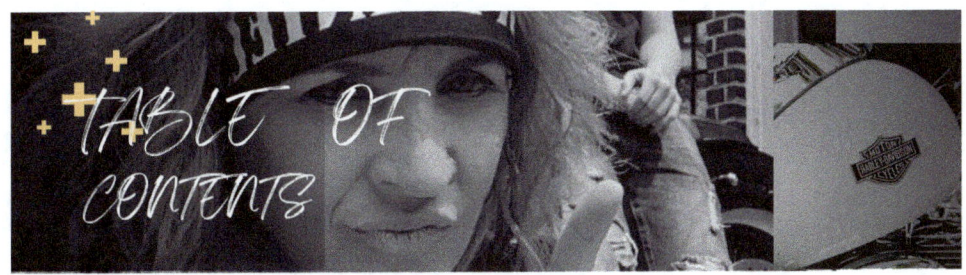

TABLE OF CONTENTS

PART IV: FIRE WE CARRY

15. Mothers, Matriarchs & the Fire We Carry........ 167
16. Brotherhood & Betrayal 176
17. The Ride That Heals 185
18. Legacy in Motion 191

FINAL CHAPTER
Never Just a Passenger 199

CLOSING ROADS
Now It's Your Turn 203
The Final Ride 204

♥ Legacy Reflection Chapter 205
Dear Younger Me 208

♥ The Patch Isn't Just His. It's Ours Too. 209
What You Might Have Missed 210
Final Affirmation Page 211
HelKat's Translator Booth 212
Dedication 217

―――― HELKAT LEGACY CO. ――――

BORN ON THE BACK OF A BIKE

"Some kids grow up in playrooms. I grew up in clubhouses."

I didn't grow up in a quiet house with bedtime stories and gentle lessons whispered at night.
I grew up with the roar of engines shaking the walls and men who spoke in code instead of comfort.
The first lullaby I ever heard was a Harley idling in the driveway.
My first classroom? The backroom of a clubhouse where loyalty was currency, respect was earned, and weakness was hunted down like prey...

───── HELKAT LEGACY CO. ─────

———— HELKAT LEGACY CO. ————

PART I
WHY NOW

"I was raised by engines,
by the roar of the road,
by lessons written in blood and loyalty."

**I wasn't born to sit pretty.
I was born to fight, to ride,
and to tell the story no one else dares.**

Because our daughters are watching us to see
what strength looks like when life falls apart.
Because we can't wait for the world to change, we
have to start with our own stories.
I am writing this book now because I've survived
just enough to finally tell the truth. And I hope it
lights the way for someone else who still thinks
she's too far gone.

CHAPTER 1:
BORN INTO THE ROAR

"Survival wasn't optional. It was the law."

I'm Helen, though in this world I go by HelKat. My story isn't pretty or polished, and I'm not here to offer you a Hallmark version of biker life. My childhood soundtrack? The clink of beer bottles and laughter carrying menace and love in equal measure.

This book is for the ones who know what it feels like to stand on the edge of two worlds: the ones who've been underestimated, silenced, or told to sit pretty while men handle the "real business." It's for the women who carry scars, who've held down families and brothers, who've learned to survive when survival wasn't guaranteed. And it's for curious outsiders, the readers who've only seen our world through TV shows, tabloids, or half-truths because what you think you know about biker culture barely scratches the surface.

I've battled cancer, lupus, and multiple sclerosis. I've buried brothers and carried sisters. I've walked the tightrope of being a woman in a world that doesn't hand you power, you take it, or you don't survive. My feminism didn't come from books; it was forged with exhaust fumes, back patches, and the sacred silence of the road.

Behind the patch, you find more than violence and rebellion, you find honor, sisterhood, heartbreak, and resilience. You find women like me, who aren't just "Ol'Ladies" in the background but warriors, healers, and voices that refuse to be erased.

So, if you're reading this looking for glamorized gangland fantasy keep flipping channels. This story isn't Sons of Anarchy. This is my truth, raw and unapologetic. And if you're the kind of reader who craves authenticity, who wants to understand how loyalty can both save and destroy you, then sit back in your chair and keep reading.

Because I'm about to tell you what it really means to live behind the patch.

"Freedom don't ask permission."

Where the Story Starts, But Not Where It Ends
I'm not your textbook feminist. I didn't come to this through lectures or literature. I came to it on city streets and broken nights. My feminism is forged in fire and fueled by freedom, the freedom to ride my own bike, build my own empire, and speak my truth even if my voice shakes. It's not about rejecting the patch, it's about redefining what it means to wear one.

And I'm not the only one. A lot of women I know are doing the same, rewriting the rules as they ride. Shifting gears not only on your chrome beast but in society as a whole. Think of your journey as a spunky mechanic revving up the dusty old ideals of feminism and rebellion, swapping out outdated parts for something with a bit more kick. Some may say I am not just a biker chick; but one that is handing out the wrenches, leading a cultural pit stop.

This isn't your grandma's memoir, unless your grandma rides a Harley and drops kickass feminist slogans between shots of tequila. This ride isn't about gentle curves or scenic routes, it's a full-throttle, witty sprint through the shifting landscapes of identity and defiance.

Because when you grow up with instability, and blood from the corner, the streets don't hand out diplomas, just scars. I came into it with calloused hands, second chances, and street lessons dressed in watching shooting, coming home to street lights and the smell of the laundry mat.

I was born into the wind, before I ever threw a leg over a Harley. Before I knew what loyalty or betrayal really felt like.

The wind and biker parties taught me first.

In biker life, nothing's handed to you. Trust is currency earned. Respect comes with a price. And survival? Well, survival is your non-negotiable admission ticket.

I grew up watching men with denim vest on their backs and women with steel in their spines. I learned early that silence wasn't safety, it was strategy. That keeping your eyes open could mean the difference between belonging and being swallowed whole.

While other kids were learning how to play nice, I was learning how to read a room, how to size up a man by the way he held his smoke, how to sense betrayal before it even had a name.

There were no soft landings, no training wheels. Childhood didn't coddle me; it toughened me. Loyalty wasn't a slogan, it was a blood oath. Respect isn't politeness, it's survival. And if you don't learn fast, you get burned, sometimes literally.

I was raised by the streets and men who measured worth in determination and by women who carried more weight than anyone gave them credit for, I'm who I am because of that. I had to learn to be proud of that.

And if you want to know who I am, start right here.
Because every scar from that road still speaks.

I spent years sitting back, watching, listening, learning what not to do. Who not to trust.
Every "no" I said was a battle.

Ride harder, speak louder and still carry yourself with just enough grace to not get labeled as trouble. Somehow, I still earned the name "HelKat" along the way.

Every decision to walk away from what I didn't understand yet, that was survival.

Because when you grow up with instability, the streets become your school.
And survival mode becomes your default setting.
I watched women lose everything: their homes, their men, their jobs, their dignity. Good women. Smart women. Tough women who just didn't get the same chance to breathe. Or who gave everything to someone who didn't deserve it. I told myself; I would not be one of them.

That was my first promise; protect what's mine. And before anything else, that meant me.
> **My body.**
> **My voice.**
> **My damn right to choose.**

This also implied that I wouldn't depend on a man for my well-being; I was determined to take care of myself. I stopped seeking someone to complete me and instead began fighting like hell to become whole on my own.

I got my ass into a dropout prevention program. I graduated. I broke the damn cycle.
Everything began to shift when someone finally saw past the walls I'd built. I found a mentor who saw me, not just the girl on the edge of everything. Someone who showed me I could speak up, stand tall, and wear my grit like a badge. Someone who taught me that grace isn't weakness, it's control. It's deciding when to show up loud and when to let silence speak louder.

That was the moment I felt myself change.
That's when the wind shifted from something I ran from to something I rode into.
And that wind? It still whispers to me every time I ride.

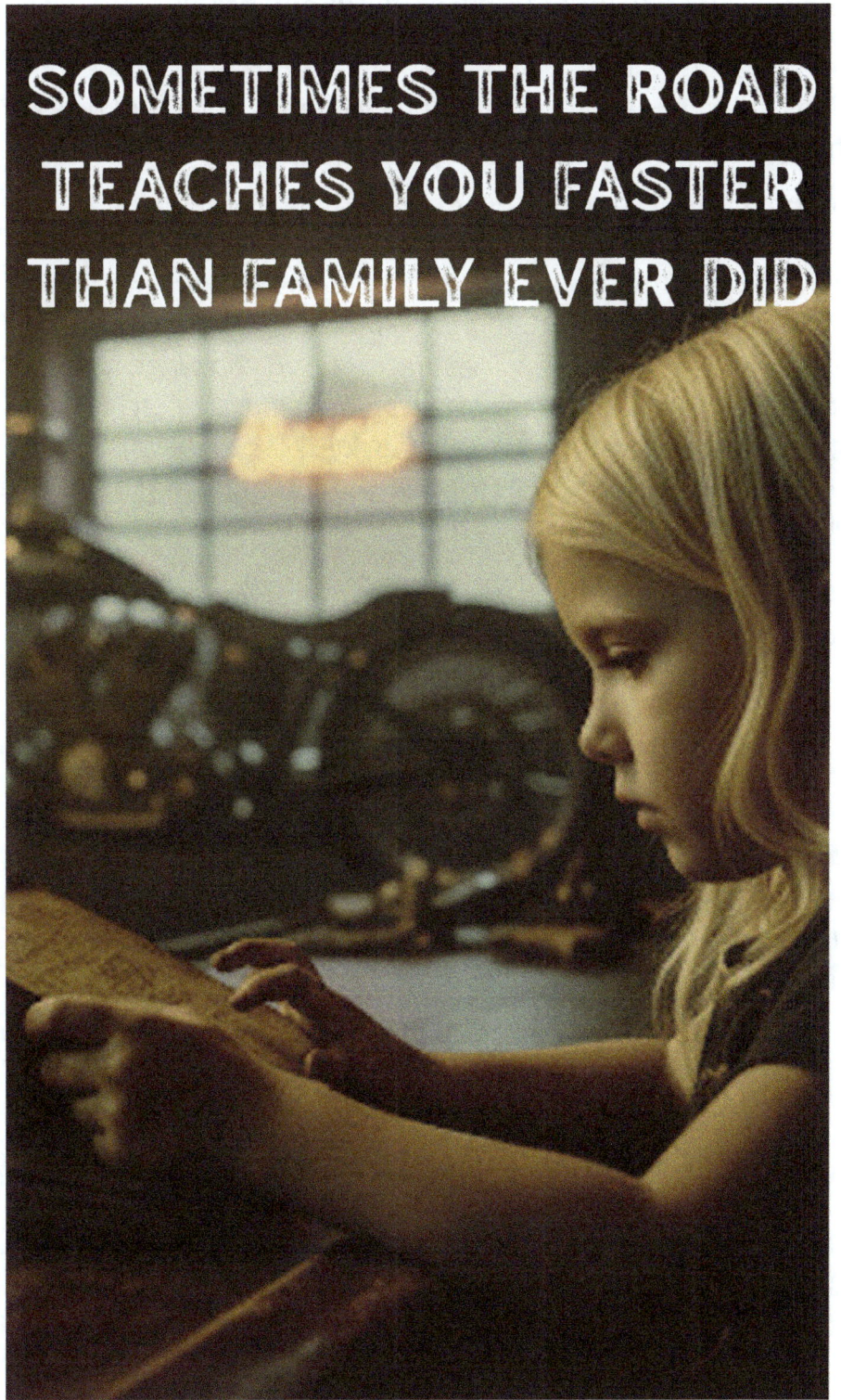

Chrome, Chaos, and the Club Code

Let's clear the air right from the jump: they're motorcycle clubs, folks, not gangs. If that tidbit's already got your knickers in a twist, this book might not be your cup of tea.

I'm not here to sprinkle sugar on anything. Forget what the media, the government, or your Aunt Karen at Sunday brunch think biker culture is about. This world has its own unwritten codes and values that demand respect.

As a woman in this scene, I've encountered challenges and secrets that would make most people's heads spin. It's shocking how often our tales get tucked away. But trust me, we're more than just leather jackets and roaring engines; we're all about honor, loyalty, and soul-stirring bonds.

I want every woman out there to hear this loud and clear: your voice matters, scars and all. Your journey is important. Whether you're navigating the club life, battling illness or trauma, or just reinventing yourself, embrace who you are. You don't need anyone's nod to live boldly and carve your own path.

Let me share a personal story. I remember a time when I was just a teenager, sitting on the back of my dad's bike. We were riding through the countryside, the wind in my hair, and the sun setting behind us. It was a moment of pure freedom, one that made me understand why this lifestyle was so important to him and eventually, to me. It was more than just the ride; it was about feeling alive and part of something bigger.

Let's bust those myths wide open and reveal the true spirit of biker culture. Because I've walked the walk. I was born into this life. And believe me, it's a tangled web. We've all heard the tales. Guns, drugs, bodies in the woods. Hollywood laps that stuff up.

But you know what doesn't make the 11 o'clock news?

It's the countless times these clubs have rallied around one of their own, raising money for a member in need or showing up in force to support a community cause. Those are the unsung stories I want to tell, the ones that truly capture what it means to be part of this world.

Behind the leather and chrome is a vibrant brotherhood and sisterhood, built on loyalty and unforgettable adventures. It's in these moments that kindness takes the spotlight. A convoy of bikers delivering toys to children during the holidays, or organizing a charity ride to support a local family in need. It's all about the bonds forged on the open road, where the thunder of engines is matched by the warmth of camaraderie.

These clubs often get a bad rap, their stories skewed by sensationalism. But among them are individuals who dedicate their lives to making a positive difference. They're mentors to the young, protectors of the vulnerable, and pillars of their communities. Their tales are rich with resilience, compassion, and a fierce commitment to one another.

So, let's peel back the layers and look beyond the stereotypes. Let's celebrate the everyday heroes who wear their patches with pride and honor. Their stories deserve to be told. Not as footnotes, but as vibrant, exciting chapters in everday life.

When they roll up to a fundraiser or a community event, they bring with them not just the rumble of their bikes but a spirit of hope and action. Each ride is a testament to their belief in the power of coming together, that by banding together, they can make a difference, no matter how big or small.

In a small community, there's the patched-up guy who always lends a hand. He once bought groceries for a single mom living down the street, proving that kindness still exists. Then there's the club that came together to raise five grand for a kid fighting cancer.

You can count on the brothers, too. They're the ones who show up at your funeral and help during fundraisers. When tough times hit, you'll find them on your front porch, ready to stand by you. It's moments like these that remind us of the values we share, the rules we live by in our little world.

These heartwarming gestures may seem simple, but they make a huge difference. Through challenges and confessions, this tight-knit group thrives because of its devotion to honor and support one another. It's not just about being part of something; it's about creating lasting bonds that are often forgotten in today's busy life. Yeah, there's chrome and chaos, but there's also "code". And that code? It matters. The motorcycle club scene, as we know it today grew out of the wreckage of World War II. Veterans came home looking for adrenaline, brotherhood, and a way to feel alive again. And they found it in the saddle of a Harley, rumbling down an open road with other men who understood what it meant to survive.

These weren't criminals, they were soldiers turned riders, looking for family in a world that had moved on without them. A lot of people don't know the history, therefore don't understand the bond or the code of respect that is vowed.

Even today, new members join, drawn by the allure of belonging to something greater than themselves. They learn the stories, adopt the values, and contribute their own chapters to this ongoing narrative.

The Patch of Identity

Wearing my own "patch" means embracing every part of who I am. Just like motorcycle riders wear their patches to show off their journeys, my patch tells the story of my life, each challenge I've faced and overcome is stitched into it. It's a reminder that I'm not just another face in the crowd; I have unique experiences that shape me.

When I see myself wearing this patch, I feel proud. It stands for courage and strength. It reminds me that even when things got tough or felt unbelievable, I kept going. There were times I felt lost or forgotten, but each patch signifies how far I've come against all odds.

My patch also connects me with others who understand what it's like to be unconventional. We share values and passions that go beyond what society expects from us. Shared bond creates a sense of honor and belonging, like we are all part of something bigger than ourselves.

So, wearing my patch isn't just about fashion, it is about identity. It is about celebrating the incredible person I am becoming through all my experiences, both good and bad. It is a badge of honor that says I am here, I have fought for my place, and I will keep pushing forward no matter what challenges come my way.

This environment didn't just raise me. it has claimed me. And there is no going back.

Raised in the roar, I learned survival early. But survival alone doesn't tell you who you are. For that, you need to face the myths, the ones stitched into the patch and the ones stitched into your own skin.

Chapter 1 Legacy Reflection Questions

1. What assumptions did you have about motorcycle clubs before reading this chapter? How did this chapter challenge or confirm them?

2. Have you ever belonged to a group where loyalty and trust meant everything? What did that experience teach you?

3. What does 'code' mean in your life? Where do you see honor, loyalty, or structure reflected in your own values or community?

Write your truth

1. What was the first moment you realized you had to protect yourself, emotionally or physically?

2. Who showed you what strength looked like, and how did they shape your path?

3. What promises have you made to yourself that you're still fighting to keep?

Pit Stop #1:

If you've ever wondered why female bikers get more double-takes than a cat in a motorcycle gang, it's because we're rewriting the biker manual, chapter one: 'Respect isn't optional, it's required.' Spoiler alert: The old boys' club isn't great with plot twists.

The best way to keep your engine running smoothly is to pull over, reflect, and laugh at just how bumpy this road really is.

CHAPTER 2:
THE PATCH, THE MYTH, AND THE WOMAN

"Scars are proof I survived, not signs of weakness."

The first time I realized being a girl meant something different, I was about eight years old, running around the edges of a clubhouse. A boy my age was handed a tiny leather vest, praised like he was already a soldier. I reached for it, too, but one of the women laughed and said, "Not for you, sweetheart. That's for the boys."
That stuck. Not because I wanted the vest, but because I wanted the recognition.

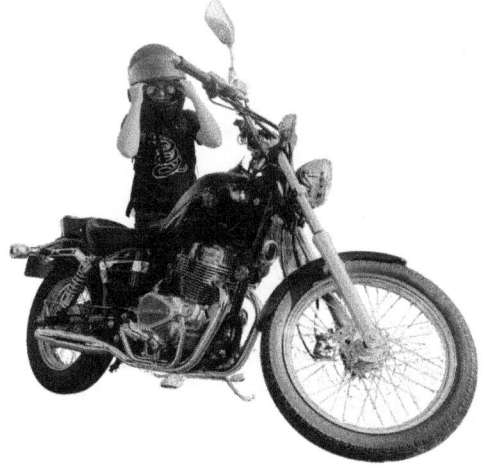

From that moment on, I grasped a lesson many of us learn too early; women in this world do not simply receive authority; we strive for it, we create it, and we fiercely protect it once it's ours.

For me, feminism wasn't born from textbooks. It emerged from the way men overlooked me until I commanded their attention. It stemmed from witnessing my mother stand her ground in chaotic bars, her voice piercing through the clamor. Being Italian, she was always loud. (Actually, she still is very loud, sorry mom)   I learned that silence could mean survival, but voicing my thoughts equated to power.

Each bruise, every illness, and every betrayal etched a singular truth deeper into my being: if I didn't claim my body, someone else would take ownership. If I didn't raise my voice, someone would work to silence it. My mother was known for her outspoken nature. I inherited that trait honestly.

That's why I write with the same fervor I ride. With unapologetic honesty, rawness, and a volume that can rattle chains. I have witnessed what occurs when women fade into the background, and I refuse to be mere wallpaper in a world I played a role in shaping.

This fight transcends my individual struggle; it belongs to all of us. For every girl told she is "too much." For every woman advised to be quiet, sit down, and accept what is offered. For every sister whose voice has been stifled. This is for you!

Many of you reading this have experienced similar moments. As women, at some point in our lives, we have all felt the gut-wrenching sting of being silenced. Of being placed second.

For those of you that need to become stronger, stay with me!

So, hear me now

You don't need permission. You don't need approval. And you don't need anyone to hand you your worth.
You were born with it.

And the day you decide to own it, the world won't just hear you, it'll never forget you.

Let's face it, sewing on a button is easy. Stitching together a life? That takes guts. More than fear (because fear is just that annoying roommate who refuses to move out). More than most will ever understand people outside the lifestyle think they know what a patch means.
TV shows. Netflix specials. True crime podcasts.
They will tell you the patch is about gangs, drugs, and violence.

But the truth?

That patch can be sacred. Or it can be a warning.
Sometimes at the same time.
For some, the patch is **protection.**
For others, it is **power.**

And for women like me, it is a **test.**
In a world where loyalty is everything and your reputation is your only defense, wearing the patch doesn't make you invincible, it makes you stand out. As a woman in this life, I have learned that strength comes from being seen and owning every part of who you are.

Every challenge I face, whether it is navigating club rules or tackling personal battles, teaches me something new about resilience. The truth can be shocking, but it also drives us forward.

It is not just about surviving; it is about thriving and finding our own way within the code of honor that governs us. We are devoted to our values and to each other. Our stories may be filled with pain, but they are also heartwarming tales of transformation and empowerment.

We carry scars proudly, knowing they tell our story. You have life scares too! You can use them to make you strong.

Now I live out loud, on my own terms no one gets to define that but me. Each word I share is an invitation for others to embrace their journey too, just like I have. This is not just my legacy; it's a roadmap for anyone ready to claim their voice and navigate the ride ahead. It marks you. And it forces you to make a choice: blend in or stand out.

I chose to stand the hell out.

Not because I wanted attention.

Because I knew I would never be a background extra in my own damn life.

I grew up watching women "earn" respect through their man, not by being seen for who they were, but by how well they played a part. They gained status by staying quiet, staying pretty, and staying in line. That kind of respect felt conditional, like it could be yanked away the moment they stopped performing. I knew I wanted something different.

Through the back of a vest. Through how well they followed rules that never seemed made for them. But I was never built for a supporting role. Even when I was an ol' lady, and I still am, I made it clear I rode my own.

I am loyal, ride-or-die, no questions asked. I am feminine, not despite the leather, but because of it. I am now fierce, not feared.

I take pride in my strength and independence, finding my own way along life's paths. My journey is filled with the sounds of roaring engines and the warmth of friends who share my passion. The open road speaks to me, reflecting my resilient spirit and natural grace. Each mile I travel is a celebration of freedom and a tribute to being unapologetically myself. My story unfolds not just through words, but in the adventures and memories captured in every ride I take.

Even back when I was just a young rebel, and still am, early in my journey, I found myself at a crossroads. I had just graduated from college, with a degree that promised stability but not much excitement. I was expected to follow a conventional path, but deep down, I knew that wasn't my destiny. I wanted to carve my own path, one where the endless road would be my guide.

So, I took a leap of faith. I sold my car, bought a motorcycle, and set out on an adventure that would change my life. My sister was skeptical, but I felt a calling to explore the world on my terms. I wanted to prove that femininity and fierceness weren't mutually exclusive.

Loyal? You bet! Ride-or-die, no two ways about it. My journey was more than just a physical one; it was a journey of self-discovery. My story isn't just told in words, it's etched in the adventures and memories of every ride I take.

As I look back on this wild adventure, I realize just how far I've traveled. I've weathered storms and basked in sunshine, tackled uphill battles and cruised through smooth sailing, and every twist and turn has been a blast. I've learned to trust my instincts and embrace the unknown, confident that the path will ultimately guide me to where I need to be. This is my story. An exciting testament to the joy of following your heart and living life on your own terms.

And nobody gets to rewrite my narrative with just three letters stitched on leather. Let's dive into what those documentaries often miss.

They often miss out on the women like me. Those who ride solo, manage their lives, and still find time to uplift their communities. That vital piece too often gets left on the cutting room floor. They fail to highlight the women who care for their families, rally to raise funds for a child battling cancer, or support a brother who laid down his bike and didn't get back up.

These biker women work harder than many men, proudly rocking both denim and lipstick.

They can fix a carburetor and mend a broken heart; all in a single weekend. It's time to shine a light on their strength and dedication; their stories deserve to be celebrated and shared.

With each ride, they prove that toughness doesn't mean sacrificing femininity. Their resilience is truly inspiring, showing that you can be passionate about your pursuits while also embracing your softer side. It's high time we honor these fierce women, as they are anything but forgotten.

So when I talk about the patch, I'm not just talking about a motorcycle club or an MC.
I'm referring to **identity**, **legacy**, and the right to be acknowledged in a world that often fails to recognize our complexity.

I no longer care how others define it.
I have already defined it for myself.

The One Percent Legacy

It is just a number 1%. Statistics. A throwaway quote from the 1940s, until it was not.

The American Motorcyclist Association supposedly said that "99% of motorcyclists are law-abiding citizens" after a wild rally in Hollister, California. Whether they actually said it or not? It doesn't even matter. Because the 1% who didn't fit the mold took that number and turned it into a movement.
A number that became an identity.
A warning.
A lifestyle.
A middle finger to anyone who said, "You don't belong."

A badge worn with pride, stitched onto leather jackets that tell stories of rebellion, freedom, and unyielding spirit. It's about carving out a space in a world that tries to box you in, about living life on your own terms and embracing the roads less traveled.

For those who wear the patch, it's not just about riding motorcycles; it's about the camaraderie, the bond forged in the shared experience of the open road. It's about the thrill of the ride, the roar of the engine, and the wind that whispers secrets of the past and promises of the future.

This legacy is passed down through generations, each

member adding their own chapter to the story, their own twist to the tale. It's a testament to resilience, a declaration of independence, and a tribute to those who dared to be different.

In a world that constantly shifts and changes, the 1% stands as a reminder that some things are timeless. Like courage, conviction, and the desire to live life on your own terms.

The Badge They Chose

For outlaw motorcycle clubs, that number became a symbol of pride. They did not care about fitting in or how suburban folks viewed them. This way of life brought challenges and confessions, often shocking but also heartwarming moments. It wasn't just about riding; it was about values and honor. Their story is huge news for those who dare to look beyond the surface.
Literally.

The 1% diamond patch became an outlaw badge of honor, sewn on vests, tattooed on flesh, inked into the legacy of biker history.

But here's the twist no one wants to talk about,
Not every 1%er is a criminal.
And not every "law-abiding" rider is squeaky clean.
This isn't black and white, it's chrome and chaos, just like the rest of club culture.

The line between right and wrong blurs, leaving only the raw essence of what it means to truly live.
These clubs are bound by more than just the pavement they ride on; they are forged in brotherhood, loyalty, and a shared understanding that life is too short to be anything but authentic.

The Misfits, The Veterans, and The Rebels

You wanna know who most early outlaw bikers were? Veterans. Survivors. PTSD-riddled men with no place to go and too much noise in their heads to sleep at night.

They weren't looking to break laws. They were looking to feel alive again, to find that adrenaline, that pack, that sense of purpose they had overseas.

And when the world rejected them, they made their own world.

One with rules. Brotherhood. Hierarchy. Respect.

One where you could lose everything, your cut, your patch, your life, if you violated the code.

So yeah, the 1% lifestyle had risks. But for some? It was the only place that felt real.

The bonds they form are often unbreakable, tested time and again by loyalty, sacrifice, and the ever-present threat of danger. These early outlaw veterans, resilient and determined, are the unsung heroes of the biker world, often holding the fabric of the club together through sheer determination and an unyielding spirit.

Outside the club, life is a constant balancing act. Members juggle the demands of the road with the responsibilities of family and work, striving to maintain a semblance of normalcy amidst the chaos. They are fathers, mothers, sons, and daughters, each with a story that transcends the leather and chrome of their chosen lifestyle.

For those on the inside, the club is both a refuge and a crucible. It's a place where the past mingles with the present, where scars are worn as badges of honor, and where every ride is a reminder of the freedom they fought so hard to claim. While the world may view them with suspicion or awe, within their ranks, they find acceptance, understanding, and a shared purpose that makes every mile worth the journey.

In the end, the motorcycle club isn't just an escape; it's a testament to the enduring human spirit, a celebration of life on one's own terms, and a family forged in the fires of adversity and adventure. It's a gritty world where politics and power play huge roles, and strict rules and a chain of command are respected. For these veterans, the club offers a sense of purpose and belonging, a place where they can feel alive again.

Living the Label (But Not Always Loving It)

Here is the part outsiders don't get: the 1%er life is not some nonstop party of guns, girls, and glory.

Life in the motorcycle club is tough and full of challenges. It's not just about riding; it's a gritty world were politics and power play huge roles. There are strict rules to follow, a chain of commands that everyone respects, and expectations hanging over your head like a dark cloud. The unwritten laws can be more confusing than any legal code you might find in a courthouse.

For women in this world, known as "Ol' Ladies," the struggle is even more intense. They have their own set of responsibilities and must navigate through the complexities of love and devotion while staying true to the club's values. It is heartwarming yet shocking to see how they thrive despite being forgotten by many outside the biker community.

Confessions shared among them reveal deep connections forged under immense stress.

Each day brings new stops and drives into unknown territories, testing their strength and determination. And when big news breaks, the ripple effects can change everything. In this life, it is all about finding a way to fit in while holding onto who you are at your core.

And the truth is, not every patch holder wanted the 1% life, some just wanted to ride. But when you are part of a club that claims that label, you inherit all the baggage, whether you earn it or not.

I have known club members who were hardworking mechanics, business owners, and family men, guys who wore the patch but also showed up for PTA meetings and church fundraisers. I have also seen patch holders spiral into chaos, addiction, and violence because of the pressure of living that outlaw legend broke them from the inside out.

And in both cases, the world judged them the same.

Modern-Day Misunderstandings

These days, the 1% diamond still gets attention, especially from law enforcement. Wear it, and you are marked. Tracked. Monitored. Stereotyped.

Sometimes that scrutiny is deserved.

Other times? It is just another way the system punishes men for building a brotherhood outside the rules.

You would be surprised how many so-called "bad guys" are doing better than most elected officials.

I have seen men pull over on the highway to help families in need. They do not always seek attention for good deeds, like when they quietly donate to bikers who lost their parents. At events, I've watched them step in to protect women when security failed to notice. These moments show how much they care and uphold their own rules of honor.

Despite the challenges they face, these acts are heartwarming reminders that kindness still thrives in unexpected places.

A Complicated Legacy

Even when the road is rough, these acts are fiery reminders that resilience and compassion are alive and thriving in every corner. But where's the recognition? The stories of their triumphs often go untold.

So, what's our legacy? Let's redefine it: It's tangible. It's hard-earned. It's often underestimated.

It's not just a badge; it's a crucible, a commitment, a challenge, and a calling entwined. It's not just a patch, it's a pressure cooker, a promise, a prison, and a purpose all rolled into one.

You don't join this sisterhood on a whim. You don't wear its emblem without understanding the weight it carries. And you certainly don't keep it without proving your mettle over and over.

But maybe, just maybe, it's time we start telling the whole story of our legacy.
Not just the struggles. Not just the headlines. But the lives. The legacies. The intricate, powerful truths behind the label.

For the men, you don't join a 1% club on a whim. You don't wear that diamond without consequences. And you sure as hell don't keep it unless you've proven yourself ten times over.

But maybe, just maybe, it's time we start telling the full story of that 1%.

Not just the felonies.
Not just the headlines.
But the lives. The legacies. The complicated truths behind the label.

The act of claiming one's identity is significant, but maintaining it in the face of personal adversity is an even more formidable task. It is a battle for which no patch can prepare you, yet it is one worth fighting for, as it ultimately leads to a more profound understanding of oneself and one's place in the world.

Transforming challenges into lessons also involves letting go of the notion that obstacles define who we are. Instead of feeling defeated when things don't go according to plan, view them as chances to explore new directions and possibilities. Just as the fearless women who ride motorcycles defy societal norms and stereotypes, you too can break free from limitations and embark on the journey to write your own story, unbound by external expectations.

Chapter 2 Legacy Reflection Questions

1. What does "the patch" symbolize to you, personally, culturally, or emotionally?

2. How have you claimed your own space in a world that did not offer it willingly?

3. What myths or labels have you had to challenge to stay true to yourself?

4. What does the phrase "1%" mean to you after reading this chapter? Has your understanding changed?

5. Have you ever been misunderstood or stereotyped because of how you look or who you associate with?

6. Do you believe people can live outside the system and still live with honor? Why or why not?

CHAPTER 3: STORM-BORN SURVIVAL - THE ROAD TO REDEMPTION

"Every mile forward was bought with pain I don't regret."

My body has been my fiercest battleground. Cancer. Lupus. Multiple sclerosis. Each one hit me like a rival gang, showing up uninvited, demanding a piece of me I wasn't ready to give.

People talk about strength like it's a choice. It isn't. It's what's left when every other option is gone.

I remember sitting in a chemo chair, fluorescent lights buzzing above, poison dripping into my veins while I tried to picture the open road. My skin was pale, my hair thinning, my hands shaking. But in my mind, I was gripping handlebars, wind in my face, and the engine under me. That vision is what kept me breathing.

Later, when I was strong enough, I climbed back on a bike with a body stitched together by scars and steel. My joints screamed with every mile, but the wind drowned out the pain. That first rally after treatment wasn't just a ride, it was a resurrection. People saw a woman on a Harley. What they didn't see was the warrior dragging three illnesses behind her like chains, refusing to let them win.

Here's the outlaw truth, illness doesn't just wreck your body. It messes with your identity. It steals your reflection, rewrites your limits, and tries to convince you you're broken. But every time I thought my body had taken something from me, I found something fiercer inside myself.

I was never strong. I was surviving. And there's a difference. Survival is crawling out of the fire even when the flames take half your skin. Survival is strapping back on your boots when your legs don't want to hold you. Survival is raising three daughters while your own body is falling apart and refusing to let them see you quit.

The diseases taught me something this lifestyle never could, strength isn't about proving you can bleed. It's about proving you'll still ride after the bleeding stops.

Here's My Truth,

I may not have power over what my body takes from me, but I absolutely have control over what I offer in return. And I choose to speak out **instead of remain silent. Every. Single Time.**

I was just a girl when I touched a cut for the first time. It was thrown over a chair, still warm from the back it had rested against, smelling of sweat, smoke, and road.

To me, it wasn't just a jean jacket. It was weight. It carried stories stitched in thread I couldn't yet read, nights of loyalty, secrets, debts, and blood. Men treated it like scripture. They'd rather lose a limb than lose their patch.

I traced the stitch with my small fingers, reverent and curious, until a hand grabbed mine and yanked me back. "You don't touch what you haven't earned," he growled.

I didn't argue, but I never forgot that moment. The cut wasn't just clothing. It was power. It was belonging. And one day, I swore, no one would tell me I hadn't earned my place behind the patch.

In my life, there are incredible women who lift me up like a motorcycle crew revving their engines together. Each of them adds their own distinct spark: Sarah's infectious laughter, Lisa's profound wisdom, and Mia's unwavering courage. Together, they create a friendship that resonates far beyond words.

Sarah, whose laughter can light up the darkest days; she reminds me that joy is worth chasing, no matter how tough things get. Then there's Lisa, always ready with wise advice and encouragement when I'm feeling lost or unsure about my path. I also think of Mia, who has this fierce courage. When I see her take risks and follow her passions, it inspires me to push through my own fears. These women are not just friends; they are heroes in my story, helping me embrace my true self and strive for greatness.

Supporting them is equally important. I want to celebrate their victories, big or small, because every win deserves recognition. Whether it's cheering them on during tough times or simply being there to listen, I know these acts strengthen our bond. It's all about creating a space where we can share our dreams without judgment.

By lifting each other up, we become an unstoppable force, much like those legendary motorcycle crews who ride through life together.

You can take the patch off a man's back, but you can't take the code out of his soul.

In the world of motorcycle clubs, your cut, that sleeveless denim or leather vest, isn't just clothing. It's armor. It's history. It's a walking résumé of who you are, who you ride for, and what you've survived.

Patches tell stories, and in this world, every thread matters.

Family-based MCs

There's a distinct difference between outlaw motorcycle clubs and family-based MCs and I've seen both sides up close. I've stood shoulder to shoulder with riders who wore the rebel badge with pride, and I've shared meals, and mission runs with MCs that felt more like family than my own blood. Too often, people outside the life lump every patch wearer into the same stereotype: lawless, dangerous, disconnected from society. But for many of us, that couldn't be further from the truth.

Yes, some clubs were born from rebellion. Outlaw doesn't always mean criminal, it often just means choosing to live outside the mainstream. But what the public misses is how many clubs are built on service, loyalty, and raising the next generation of riders with honor.

Family-based MCs or organizations prioritize community. We raise funds, support local causes, and raise our kids to respect the road and the people on it. This life teaches discipline, tradition, and love that runs deeper than blood.

"Just because we ride outside the lines doesn't mean we ride without rules."

What's a Cut "Jacket", You Ask?

Alright, listen up, rookies! Here's the scoop. The mighty "cut" is short for cut-off, a decked-out vest usually born from denim or leather. This bad boy is where the club's colors, a.k.a. patches, are sewed on with precision and pride. Each patch is like a badge of honor, telling tales of purpose, position, and pride.

When you spot someone rocking a cut (Jacket), you're not just witnessing a fashion statement! Nope! you're seeing commitment, camaraderie, and sometimes a sprinkle of conflict or harmony. But above all, it's a badge of purpose.

Every patch spins a yarn, and if you've got the know-how, you can read a man's story right off his back.

In the biker realm, respect is earned, one stitch at a time. The cut is more than leather or denim. It's a whole language. It's not just fashion; it's identity. It's history you can wear.

Colors. Rockers. Patches. Each symbol means something, and if you don't know what you're looking at, you might get yourself in trouble.

You don't buy a cut, you earn it. And when you wear it? You'd better know what the hell it means.

Understanding the Structure of a Traditional Club Patch

A top rocker tells you about territory. A bottom rocker tells you allegiance. The center patch? That's the soul of the club.

Here's a breakdown of a classic club patch configuration. I learned early, never touch another biker's cut. That vest is sacred. You don't mess with it, not if you value your teeth.

A traditional club patch isn't just decoration. It's a language. At the top is the rocker with the club's name. Simple enough.

Below that sits the center patch. The logo, the mascot, the symbol everyone recognizes. That piece is sacred. You don't touch it, don't joke about it, don't earn it halfway. It means something, and everyone who knows the culture knows that.

Then there's the small MC patch. Short for Motorcycle Club. Usually tucked on the right side. It's understated, but it carries weight. And finally, the bottom rocker. That's the territory. The place the club claims, protects, or represents. Some clubs wear it loud. Others don't wear one at all. That's not an accident, it's strategy.

To outsiders, it's just thread. To those who understand, it's a résumé, a warning, a family tree, and a promise all stitched together. These patches don't announce themselves. They don't need to. The message is already clear to the people it's meant for.

For outsiders, these symbols may seem cryptic, but for those within, they are a living history. Each patch tells a story, and each story is a chapter in the epic saga of the club. Whether it's a tale of triumph or trial, joy or sorrow, each patch is a piece of the larger narrative, contributing to the legacy that members carry with pride.

As you ride, those patches become a part of you, etched into your soul as deeply as the miles traveled together. And with every new journey, they continue to collect stories, adding layers of depth and meaning.

The Power of the Back Patch

Wearing a club's colors on your back is a sacred act. It says, "I belong." It also says, "I will protect this club with everything I've got."

The back patch is not a fashion accessory. It's a declaration. It comes with responsibility. And it comes with risk.

If you're caught wearing club colors you haven't earned or pretending to be part of a club when you're not, you're not just being disrespectful. You're being reckless. Because in this world, colors are sacred, and poser patches get dealt with. I'll never forget the first time I understood the weight of a patch.

I watched a brother take off his cut at a funeral and drape it over a casket. It wasn't just leather, it was loyalty laid to rest. In that moment, I understood: a patch isn't worn, it's carried. It carries you, too.

Some people think cuts are just for show. But in this world, they're contracts. Oaths. If a man breaks his, the whole club bleeds for it.

Patches Tell the Story

The colors and designs symbolize belonging and history, marking the wearer's journeys and battles. In a world where trust and loyalty are extremely important, these patches serve as a visual language, respected by those who understand their importance.

Oh, honey, let me tell you! These patches have more stories than this ol' lady's got years. I've seen them all. Some flaunt bold claims like "1%" for that rebellious spirit, or "Property of" to declare a love as fierce as a biker's grip on the throttle. They stir the pot, they do. But others, like those precious memorial patches, softly whisper tributes to the ones we lost along the way. Each patch has a voice too. Some scream with the ferocity of a Harley on the open road, others murmur like wind through the trees, but none are mute. We ware our stories on our sleeves, literally, because the patches are more than fabric. They are badges of honor, and whispers of the heart.

For those who live life on two wheels, patches aren't souvenirs. They are the backbone of a brotherhood and sisterhood that doesn't ask for much but expects everything. Every patch tells the world you've earned your place. These colors are a handshake at the gas station, a nod across the bar, a shield against anyone who doesn't get what it means to ride for something bigger than yourself. Out here, respect isn't given. It's proven, mile after mile.

Step into any biker gathering and you'll notice it, even if you can't quite name it yet. The patches start talking before anyone opens their mouth. Take the 1% patch. It doesn't need a speech. It signals a choice to live outside the usual lines. Or Live Pagan, Die Pagan. Not a catchy phrase; a promise, worn where everyone can see it.

Some patches invite debate, especially from people looking in from the outside. "Property of" is one of those. It makes folks uncomfortable, mostly because they try to translate it using rules that don't quite apply here. To some, it reads as control. To others, it's loyalty claimed openly and without apology. Both readings may say something true, depending on where you're standing.

Memorial patches slow everything down. They aren't about status. They're about remembering the ones who didn't make it to the next ride, and quietly reminding everyone else not to take their time for granted. Not every patch speaks loudly, either. Some are just numbers or letters, shorthand that only means something if you already know. And if you don't, the safest move is observation, not interpretation. This isn't a culture that rewards guessing.

So, when you see a rider's back covered in stories, you're not looking at decoration. There's a learning curve to all of it, and most people outside the culture don't realize how steep it is. You don't just walk into a shop, pick out a patch, and sew it on. That's not how any of this works. The patch isn't the beginning of the story. It's more like the end of a very long first chapter.

What outsiders sometimes miss is that the patch system, for all its visual drama, is really just a way of making the invisible visible. Loyalty, rank, grief, defiance, and love. None of those things are easy to say out loud, especially in a culture that tends to distrust words anyway. A patch says it without saying it. Which is maybe why the people who wear them guard them so seriously

The Women Who Read It Too

Don't think for a second women don't understand this code. I could read a cut before I could ride a bike. I knew which clubs to steer clear of, which men had power, and which ones were just trying to look tough.

For women in this world, that knowledge is survival. You don't flirt with colors you don't understand. You don't hang on the back of just anyone's bike. You read the cut, you read the man, and you decide if he's worth your time.

Every person you encounter carries a narrative, revealed not only through their attire but also through their demeanor. They have a story and it is under what they wear as much as what they wear.

Ah, those were the days, when the notorious club would roll through town like a thunderstorm on wheels, leaving a trail of excitement and apprehension in their wake. The rumble of their engines was a signal that the wild ones had arrived, and anyone with sense knew to keep their distance, lest they be swept up in the whirlwind of leather and chrome.

My dear friend Daisy, who's been around since the early days, once shared a story that has stuck with me ever since. She reminisced about her first encounter with one of their members, and the memory seemed to twinkle in her eyes. "I was at the local diner," she began, "just enjoying my usual cup of java, when this guy strolled in. He was the epitome of the biker image. Leather vest, tattoos, the whole shebang. But it wasn't just his appearance that caught my attention; it was the way he moved, the confidence in his stride.

He had an air of assurance about him, not the least bit arrogant. I knew right then and there that he was the genuine article, the real McCoy. We ended up chatting for hours, and by the end of our conversation, I realized I had to be cautious. Sure, he was charming, but beneath that charm, I sensed a wild streak lying in wait. From that day forward, I learned to always trust my instincts about who to engage with and who might be best left alone."

Daisy's tale left an indelible mark on me, serving as a solid reminder that sometimes it's not just about reading the patch they wear, but understanding the person beneath it. Her story, woven with nostalgia and a hint of adventure, often comes to mind when I think about those days gone by.

The Tattooed Identity

If patches are your uniform, tattoos are your dog tags.
Tats might show club initials, logos, slogans, or that infamous 1% diamond. But like the patch, club ink must be earned. You don't tattoo the name of a club on your body unless you've bled for it. Lived for it. Proven you won't run when things get hot.

And if you betray the club after getting that tattoo? Let's just say there are methods for removal, most of them painful.

I remember a particular day vividly. My man decided to get a tattoo that would seal his bond with the club. As he sat in the chair, I watched the artist work, each stroke of the needle a testament to the loyalty he held dear. The design wasn't just ink on skin; it was a commitment to the life he had chosen and to the brothers who stood by him. As the image took shape, I felt a swell of pride mixed with a touch of apprehension. This was more than a tattoo it was a promise to stand firm no matter what came our way.
For those on the outside, this might be hard to understand.

But for us, it's as clear as the lines etched into his flesh. The club became my anchor in the storm, a brotherhood bound not just by ink and denim, but by shared experiences and unspoken understandings. Every mark on his skin is a pledge, a promise that we'll stand by our brothers and sisters, come what may. In this tight-knit world, respect is earned with every mile ridden and every challenge faced together. Watching him get that tattoo was a reminder of the strength and commitment that binds us all.

It was a rite of passage, a visible testament to the sacrifices made and the loyalty pledged. Each member of our club carries with them a story inked onto their skin, a narrative written in shades of black and blue, colors that signify resilience and unity.

As he rose from the chair, the fresh tattoo gleaming under the dim light, I knew this was a moment that would linger in our memories. It was a bond that couldn't be broken by time or distance.

In our world, these tattoos are more than just art; they're a declaration of who we are and what we stand for. They tell a story of battles fought and victories won, of nights spent riding under the stars and days filled with laughter. It's a tradition that connects us to those who came before and will guide us into the future, a legacy etched in skin, living and breathing with each heart that beats beneath it.

When a Patch Is Taken

Stripping a man of his patch is one of the most brutal things that can happen in club culture. It's a public mark of dishonor. A symbolic death. In some clubs, it's followed by an actual beating, or worse.

Because once you betray the patch, you betray the brotherhood. And there are consequences.

I've seen men removed with grace. I've also seen them removed with blood.

But either way? The patch never leaves quietly. The cut matters. But so does what's underneath it. Some men wear the cut but don't live the code. They chase clout, not loyalty. And when shit hits the fan, they fold.

The real ones? Their cut is just the outside layer. You strip it away, and the loyalties are still tattooed in their bones. That's the difference between wearing a cut and carrying legacy.

At times, patches are removed for a designated period, allowing for the possibility of regaining membership. In some cases, they are taken permanently, leaving no chance for reentry. Occasionally, opportunities for returning to a prospect and relearning are provided.

Taking away a man's patch is one of the most severe blows in club life, it's a public humiliation, a shattering of the spirit. This act can sometimes escalate into violence or worse. Betraying the patch means betraying the brotherhood, and the repercussions are swift and severe.

I've seen men leave with dignity, while others have been forcibly removed amid chaos. I recall a guy named Mike from my early days in the club. He was older, had been around longer, and had seen more than most of us. Mike always seemed untouchable, like he was part of the club's foundation.

But then rumors started about him cutting deals behind the clubs back. It was hard to believe, and harder to watch when the truth came out. The day they took Mike's patch, it felt like the air had been sucked out of the county.

Regardless, the patch never departs in silence. The cut is vital, but so is the soul beneath it. Some wear it for show, not for truth. They chase shadows, not loyalty. And when chaos erupts, they crumble.

The true ones? Their cut is just skin-deep. Strip it away, and their loyalty remains etched in their bones. That's the essence of wearing a cut versus living a legacy.

Watching Mike struggle afterward, it was clear that without the patch, he was lost. He tried to make amends, but some betrayals are too deep to mend. It was a lesson for all of us. A reminder that the patch only represents what's truly inside.

When my man came home in a plain jacket, my heart clenched with a mix of concern and quiet understanding. I knew the significance of the patch and what it meant to wear one. Its absence spoke volumes, telling a story of change, of something lost and left behind.

I found myself letting out a soft sigh, acknowledging the weight he carried without it. There was no need to bombard him with questions; in the world of clubs, actions and circumstances often speak louder than words.

I offered him a comforting presence with a warm meal and a calming embrace, giving him the space to share his story when he felt ready. My loyalty wasn't tied to the patch he once wore but to the man he was beneath it. I stood by him, unwavering, knowing that while the jacket might be plain, our bond and my support were steadfast and enduring.

More Than Colors, It's Culture

To the outside world, it might look like a bunch of angry dudes in leather or denim vests. But to us? Those vests are sacred. The patches sewn on them are years of pain, protection, and life lived.

Most can spot another rider's cut from a mile away. I remember once pulling into a rural gas station and clocking a man's bottom rocker before he even got off his bike. His patch told me he rode with a rival crew known for handling things rough. I adjusted my tone, stayed alert, and kept the peace. That one glance told me everything I needed to know and probably saved me from a confrontation I didn't need.

You see where they're from, who they roll with, and what kind of business they're about. It gives you a scoop on whether you should show some respect or whether you should watch your six. In the MC world you don't ask what someone does.

Let's face it, life isn't always a dazzling show. Sometimes, it feels like the world crashes down, but the true test lies in how we rise from the rubble. Our scars, each a chapter in our story, echo our truths. To every woman navigating the pulse of club life, the shadows of illness, the echoes of trauma, or the winds of transformation, remember: your voice is a force, waiting to be reclaimed.

So, whether you're pushing through storms or basking in triumphs, wear your journey like a badge. Own your path, stand firm in your truth, because in this biker world, it's all about heart, and no one has the right to define yours. In the MC realm, you don't ask someone's role. You read their back. The cut isn't just fabric; it's a vow sewn in blood, and breaking it costs more than flesh.

If hospitals showed me my fragility, this life revealed my unbreakable spirit. Both types of scars, trust me, have their own tales to tell.

Chapter 3 Legacy Reflection Questions

1. Have you ever worn something that made you feel powerful or seen? What was it, and why did it matter to you?

2. How do you honor the communities or people who've shaped you?

3. What does "earning" something mean in your own life? How do you recognize that in others?

CHAPTER 4: PROSPECTING AIN'T FOR THE WEAK

"I burned down the life that burned me first."

You don't walk into a motorcycle club and grab a patch like it's a t-shirt at a merch table. You earn it. And before you earn it? You bleed for it.
That's what it means to be a prospect.

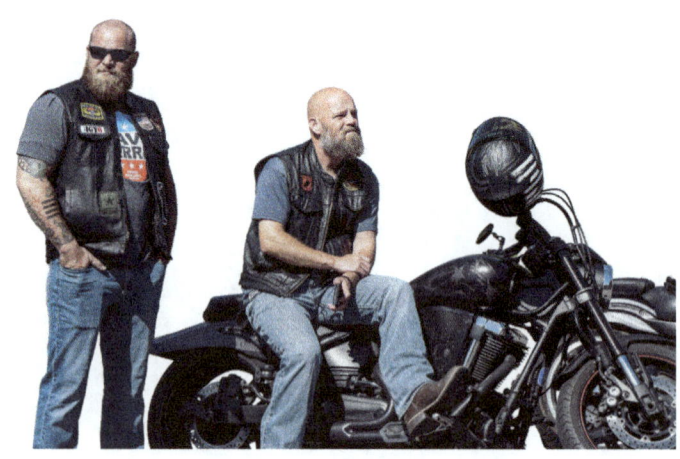

In the MC world, prospecting isn't just about joining a club. It's about proving you deserve a brotherhood that could save you or destroy you. It's not a title. It's a test. The kind that grinds you down until there's nothing left but your word and your will.

A prospect is the rookie. The one trying to earn his place. Think of it like boot camp, just louder, dirtier, and with a hell of a lot more attitude. No perks, no shortcuts. Prospects clean bikes, haul gear, run errands, and guard doors through rain and silence. They shut up and watch, because watching teaches survival. Every move matters. Every mistake echoes.

And here's the truth, **not everybody's built for it.**
Remember from chapter two; a lot of these guys started off as veterans.

Some stand in the rain all night with numb hands and empty stomachs. Some get barked at until they break. Some never come back. Because this world doesn't want the tough, it wants the proven. You don't earn a patch for showing up. You earn it for showing up when nobody else does.

Servants or Brothers?
From the outside, people say prospects are treated like servants.

But the real ones know better.

It isn't humiliation. It's trust training.

It's the question every brother asks without words:
"Will you still be there when it gets bad?"

Because in a real club, your brother's life might depend on it.

Yeah, there are some dark corners. Some outlaw clubs push too far with breaking men to own them. They make loyalty dirty, wrapping it in crime and fear so you'll never walk away. That's not loyalty. That's control.

But most clubs? They don't need to break you. They forge you. Through service. Through discipline. Through showing up when no one's clapping. That's the fire that tempers steel.

Forged in Fire

Watching a man prospect is like watching iron meet flame. Every weakness shows. Every strength is tested. I've seen good men crumble and I've seen others rise like smoke. One guy forgot to gas up the bikes before a long ride. Rookie mistake. They roasted him for weeks. But instead of sulking, he doubled down. Showed up early. Checked every tank, every time. By the end of that year, he was the one they trusted to lead the pack.

That's what prospecting does. It burns away ego until all that's left is integrity.

The Women Beside the Fire

Women don't wear prospect patches, but we have our own initiation. To accept an Ol'lady or property patch, there are rules. Most clubs require a year with an Ol'man before wearing his jacket.

We keep things moving when men falter. We fundraise, fix, feed, protect, and repair what's broken. We run toward the fire, not from it.

People tell us to "stay pretty and stay quiet." But real biker women? We guard doors, clean wounds, bury brothers, yet still show up for Sunday rides. We don't stand by, we stand with.

Not behind. Not beneath.

This life demands the same from us as it does from them. The same grace and guts to rise again. We need Commitment and understanding when we say "Yes" to wearing his jacket.

His journey is about earning his own jacket but with that he is earning patches for is lady and a commitment for his whole family.

On the road of life, resilience becomes our most trusted companion. We learn that courage isn't the absence of fear but the determination to act despite it. Every scar tells a story of battles fought and survived, each one a testament to our unwavering spirit.

The prospect grind, whether it's in the arenas of personal growth, professional ambition, or everyday survival, demands more than just perseverance. It requires a deep-seated belief in our own capabilities and the willingness to rise each time we fall. It's about crafting our own destiny, one determined step at a time, and knowing that, in the end, we are the architects of our own stories.

So we continue, fueled by the lessons of the past, ever ready to face whatever comes next with the same tenacity and grace that brought us this far.

Parallel Truths

I understand the prospect grind because I have watched and I have been apart of two ladies organizations running similar codes. I have accepted a "property" patch. I have lived it.

Prospects wrestle for their slice. Women battle for their value.

I grappled with a world relentless in questioning my value.

We're both out to prove that loyalty isn't stitched into fabric; it's forged in the steadfastness when tempers flare.

The Code of Honor

This life, club or not, runs on a code. Mine's simple,

- **Devotion** — to the people who matter, even when it's hard.

- **Respect** — starting with yourself, for without it, all else crumbles.

- **Courage** — to face down fear, even if you're the only one still standing.

That's my compass. My map through the chaos.

I didn't learn it from rules. I learned it from pain. From my father. From watching loyalty get tested in silence.

So yeah, prospecting ain't for the weak.
But neither is womanhood in this life.
We're forged in the same fire, just different flames.

And when the smoke clears, you'll know exactly who you are.
Because survival, my friend, doesn't come with a patch.
It comes with **scars that shine.**

Chapter 4 Legacy Reflection Questions

1. Have you ever had to prove yourself in a high-pressure situation? What did you learn about yourself?

2. What does loyalty look like in your world? Who has shown it to you, and who have you shown it to?

3. What's something in your life you had to earn the hard way? Was it worth it?

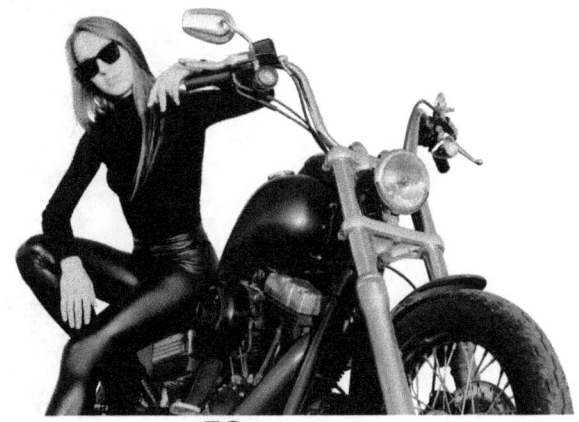

CHAPTER 5:
RAISED BY THE WIND

"Even in pieces, I ride."

In the club, brotherhood isn't just a word. It's a lifeline. It's the silent agreement that if you go down, someone's hauling you back up, no questions asked.

But let's be real, people throw the word around too easily. Brotherhood/Sisterhood isn't about drinking together or riding side by side on the open road. It's about who shows up when the road ends in fire.

I've seen it with my own eyes.

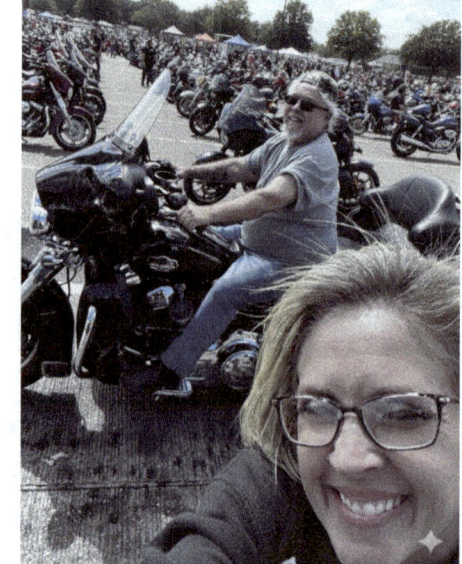

One night after a ride, a brother laid his bike down hard on a back road. Asphalt ripped him up, blood everywhere, his cut torn open. By the time I reached him, two others were already there, one ripping off his own shirt to stop the bleeding, the other calling in backup. No hesitation. No panic. Just action. That's what brotherhood looks like. Not the patches. Not the photo ops. The moments when someone's life is hanging on a thread and you don't blink before tying the knot.

That's why betrayal stings so deep in this world. Because once you've trusted someone with your life, the wound of being screwed over never really heals.

I've watched men toast to loyalty on Friday night, then throw each other under the bus by Sunday morning. And I've also watched men stand guard outside a hospital room for days, making sure no one fucked with their brother while he healed.

Hell, I can testify, with all my hospital stays, people stood guard outside my room and beside my bed. Once, when the nursing station limited visitors to two, my room was soon filled with over a dozen bikers.

Brotherhood is messy. It's sacred. And it's tested in ways outsiders will never understand.

The truth? It isn't perfect. Sometimes any relationship can let you down. Sometimes egos crack the bond. Sometimes what looks like family from the outside feels fractured on the inside. But when it's real? It's unstoppable.

Because when the storm hits, you don't need everyone. You just need the ones who won't disappear.

It's not about the patches on your back; it's about the silent promises made in the toughest times. It's about knowing that no matter the distance or the differences, the bond remains unbroken.

So, when you find that rare connection, hold onto it. Cherish it. Because in a world that's often unpredictable and harsh, true brotherhood is a refuge. A place where loyalty isn't just a word but a way of life. It's the fire that keeps you warm, the anchor that keeps you grounded, and the compass that guides you home.

A Different Kind of Upbringing

While other kids were learning their ABCs, I was learning the sound of a shovelhead engine echoing through the alley. My daddy was a dirt hog, grease under his nails, oil in his blood, and more stories in his saddlebag than most men get in a lifetime. He didn't raise me to be afraid of much. He raised me to hold my own, speak up, and ride with intention.

I still remember being five years old, my small hands wrapped around his worn t-shirt as he let me balance on the bike in the alley. He looked me dead in the eye and said, 'The road doesn't care if you're a man or a woman, it only cares if you respect it.' That line never left me.

And I've been riding ever since.

Forget ballet and playdates, I grew up at biker rallies, wrenching beside grown men and learning real-world rules no schoolbook could teach. My babysitters weren't nannies, they were tattooed brothers who taught me how to gut a deer, fire up a bonfire, and stand up to anybody who disrespected me.

By the time I was old enough to ride, I didn't need someone to hold the handlebars. I was ready to take the road head-on. Not on the back seat, on my own damn bike. My dad taught me well.

Not Just a Pretty Face

People see me now with long blonde hair, tattoos, confidence, and yeah, I'm the type to turn heads at the gas station. But don't let the pretty fool you. I have a mouth like a sailor. Like the time a guy smirked and asked whose bike I was polishing. I swung a leg over, fired it up, and left him in exhaust fumes before he could finish his laugh. Bitch, I polish my own while you dream of me polishing yours.

I'm a ride-or-die woman who speaks with volume and walks with purpose. Because being sexy isn't weakness. It's a weapon when you know who you are.

In this world? That earns your respect. You have to demand it.

Riding Through a Man's World

Let me tell you, being a strong woman in a sea of leather-clad alpha males isn't for the faint of heart. But I've been hustling in male-dominated arenas since I could clock in. I've outworked, outtalked, and outlasted more than half of them, from convenience stores to factories, farms, and even politics. I have learned a lot.

At 47, I've stared down cancer, lupus, and MS. I've raised kids, built businesses, and spoken at events where some folks didn't expect a woman to say what needed saying. But trust me, they remember me when I'm done! They don't talk over me twice. Not happening on my watch. Mistake me for being soft? Only if they're ready for some unexpected surprises. I've always got a quick-witted, sharp-tongued comeback at the ready, just waiting to be unleashed.

Once, after I finished my speech, a grizzled biker, with a beard as tough as steel, strides over to me. His arms are crossed as he grumbles, "Didn't expect to be listening to a woman tonight. But you sure shut me up." That's the kind of respect that's earned through sheer grit, not something that's just handed out like candy at a parade.

When it comes to love, I love with an intensity that's fierce and unwavering. And if I choose to stand by a man, it's because he's truly earned that place, not because he's got some imaginary leash on me.

Some women drift in and out of life like the ever-changing seasons. But me? I stay put. I build something lasting. I grow and evolve. And when I make my entrance?

I don't just show up. I arrive with an undeniable bang.

Loud, Laughing, and Leading

Yeah, I'm loud. I cuss. I dance in boots and jeans and throw back tequila with the best of 'em. But I'm also the one organizing rides, running benefits, and making sure the kids at the rally get fed and feel safe.

One year, when the food truck broke down. I raided three coolers, sparked a fire pit, and turned what could have been a dud into the most legendary cookout anyone had ever witnessed. That's respect! Not simply given, but earned with a fiery flair and a touch of creativity.

People still talk about that night, not because it was perfect, but because we made it happen anyway.

I've carried friends through addiction, loss, divorce, and burnout. I've also carried event tents, firewood, and three drunk bikers to their bunks after a poker run.
It's all part of the life.

But through it all, I ride with purpose. I live with power. And I speak with the voice of every biker woman who refuses to be tamed.

Legacy on Lock

This lifestyle raised me. But now, I'm shaping it.

I write, coach, and raise funds to create spaces for women like me, biker women with strong spirits and big dreams. We're rewriting the motorcycle myths that forget us. It's wild how many rules and values we challenge just by showing up.

We define devotion in motion. Together, we thrive in a world where our hearts honor each other and embrace the code of sisterhood.

At one ride, I watched a young woman hesitate at the edge of the lot. I handed her a helmet, said, 'Your story starts today,' and rode beside her for the first ten miles. That's the legacy I want, opening the road for the next sister.

I ride beside my man, but I stay true to myself. My boots have walked through hell and still look good doing it. We don't just face the road, we own it. We face challenges and share confessions, sometimes shocking, but always heartwarming. Each ride is a reminder of what we cherish, driving forward despite the stops along the way. This journey thrives on our resilience, making huge waves in a community where many feel forgotten.

So, when I say I was born into the wind? What I mean is... The road I have lived made me unstoppable.

It's like peeling back your skin to see what you've buried just to fit in. Many of us learn early on that certain qualities might not fit the mold of who we're "supposed" to be.   Normally we learn it in grade school.

Maybe you've hidden your passions, those wild dreams that feel too big for a world full of rules and expectations. Perhaps you've felt pressured to downplay your unique spirit, your bravery, or even those quirky traits that make you stand out.

Think about it. Society has its own twisted code, a set of unspoken rules about beauty, strength, and how we're "supposed" to be. It's messy. It's loud. It's scary and radiant and real. Commercial even put pressure on how we should look, what to wear and how to live. Most of us use filters before posting a single picture to social media.

When we dare to show up raw and unfiltered, flaws and fire included, we unlock something powerful. Because there's real freedom in owning your whole damn story.

So many times, we've been told that being pretty means being quiet or that showing courage means always being serious. But in reality, true beauty is messy and complicated,

Just like life itself. It doesn't come from fitting into someone else's idea of perfect but rather from embracing all parts of ourselves, our shiny victories as well as our gritty struggles. When we're brave enough to show up naked and real, with all our flaws and strengths laid bare, that's where magic happens. You see, it's incredible how much freedom there is in owning our stories.

They can call us Ol' Ladies all they want. But behind the patch, we are the spine that keeps the whole damn body standing.

Brotherhood isn't about who rides beside you when the sun is shining. It's about who bleeds beside you when the night turns violent.

And those are the ones I ride for.

Growing up in that world meant understanding the unspoken. And for women, the unspoken rules were sometimes heavier than the ones stitched into any patch.

Families in the biker world don't look like the ones you see on TV. They're loud, messy, patched together with duct tape and bad decisions, but they hold. Or at least, they try to. This may be why gorilla tapa was invented.

My own blood family was no exception. Love wasn't something we said much. It was something you proved or failed to. My father... that relationship was a wreck before it ever had a chance to be built.

I used to hate my old man for what he wasn't. I know that sound bad but let me explain first.

He wasn't a doctor or a lawyer, but neither where the fathers of my school friends. He wasn't clean-shaven, buttoned up, or driving some shiny new truck. He was grease-stained and road-worn, roaring up on a Harley that rattled the block. Sometimes a Mustang that coughed smoke like it was allergic to good manners. His jeans were always torn, his t-shirt reeked of oil, and those faded tattoos crawled down his forearms like warnings. He got them when he came home from war.

Maybe I hated how it made me feel. Inferior, less-than. Ashamed to admit I was his daughter.

Years later, I sat in my living room, a beer gone warm in my hand, staring at the grandfather clock that's been in our family longer than I've been alive. (Which I think my aunt now owns.) Every tick sounded like a reminder of the times I told him I didn't want to see him. Like shame was carved into seconds.

Funny how time shifts your vision.

I see him now. Not the embarrassment. Not the oil stains. But the man who held the line in his own broken way.

"Dad," I whisper to no one but the walls, "we lost years. That's on me as much as you. But I'm heading back now. Taking the long way through the mountains, just like you always said. Sixty miles an hour, no windshield, nothing between me and the truth but the wind. You were right."

Tears burned, not because I was weak, but because regret is a motherfucker when you finally own it. I wasn't better than him. I wasn't above him. I was him. And maybe the road was just another door I had to find the guts to open.

That night, I flipped on the garage light and stared at my '95 Road King. Dust dulled the chrome, grief dulled the rider. My hand brushed the seat, and I could almost feel him there. For the first time, I let myself believe that someday soon, me and Dad would take that ride together. The one we never got around to. The one that would stitch something back together in both of us.

Determined, I grabbed a rag and a bottle of polish, and began to restore the shine to the Road King. Each circular motion felt like a ritual, a way to honor the past while preparing for the future.

As the chrome began to shine again, a sense of peace washed over me. I realized that this journey wasn't just about reconnecting with Dad, but also about finding a part of myself that had been lost along the way. It was about embracing the unknown, trusting that the road would reveal its secrets and guide me to where I needed to be.

I stepped back, admiring the bike. It was ready, and so was I. Soon, we would ride together, and with every mile, a new chapter would unfold, filled with hope, healing, and the promise of what lay ahead.

And maybe Momma Betty, housebound with cancer for nearly a decade, would finally get her freedom in the sound of those pipes. Maybe she's already in God's hands, smiling while Dad steps into the next version of himself.

Because the road always leads home, if you've got the guts to follow it.

Chapter 5 Legacy Reflection Questions

1. What part of your upbringing shaped your identity the most? Was it freedom, hardship, or something in between?

2. How do you honor where you came from while still growing into who you're meant to be?

3. What does it mean to "ride your own" in life, not just on a bike, but in relationships, business, or healing?

Pit Stop #2: The Helmet Debate

Ah, helmets, our faithful companions on the road and the ultimate symbol of "I came prepared" or, depending on the biker gang, "I dare you to question my toughness." When I tugged on mine, I realized it wasn't just about protecting my head; it was about protecting a woman's right to ride without being mistaken for a careless passenger. Turns out, helmet hair might be a small price to pay for smashing the stereotype that women riders are just "along for the ride." Feminist True Fact: The helmet is both shield and subtle badge of rebellious respect.

PART II
LOVE, LOYALTY & LOSS

"Loyalty isn't tested in loud moments.
It's tested in silence,
in the choices that no one else sees."

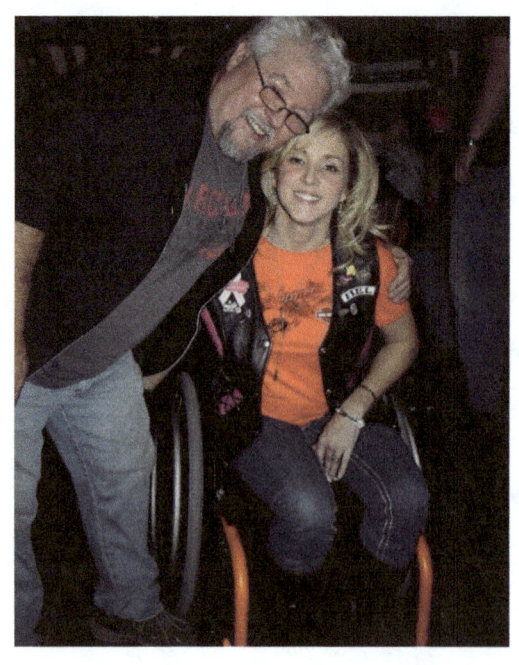

CHAPTER 6: THE WEIGHT OF AN OL' LADY

"Not every woman wears a patch, but we damn sure carry the weight."

The thing about fathers, families, even clubs, they all teach you the same hard truth. Love ain't clean, and loyalty sure as hell isn't simple. My dad wasn't perfect. Neither was I. But what stitched us together wasn't polish. It was the road, the roar, and the understanding that scars tell the real story.

That's the same lesson I learned in the clubhouse. Respect wasn't handed to me because of a last name or bloodline. It was earned. Fought for. Bled for.

The patch? That little square of fabric everybody sees as a fashion statement? It's a whole different beast. It carries weight, law, and price tags people outside will never understand.

Which is why the next chapter isn't about chrome or leather. It's about the cost. The price you pay to wear it. And the ways women like me learned to carry it without ever getting stitched in.

The world has a way of simplifying biker women into stereotypes: the background eye candy, the girl on the back seat, the "property of" tag like we're accessories instead of flesh and blood.

But the truth? Ol' Ladies are the backbone. We're the ones holding families together when the men are too broken, too drunk, or too blinded by the next ride. We're the voices of reason when the club threatens to rip itself apart. And we're the ones who shoulder loyalty without needing a patch to prove it.

I've watched women pull together fundraisers that kept the lights on for widows. I've seen them cook for fifty people on nothing but grit and donated groceries. I've seen them pull a man out of a bar fight, bloodied and swinging, and still manage to get him home safe.

I remember one night, a brother stumbled into the clubhouse wrecked from grief. His ol' lady didn't hesitate, she took his keys, poured his drink down the drain, and told him to sit his ass down. No one argued with her. Not even the men who outranked her. That's the power of a real ol' lady.

But let's not sugarcoat it. Sometimes the title comes with chains. "Property Of" patches can weigh heavy, especially when respect gets twisted into control. I've seen women lose themselves in the role, disappear into someone else's shadow, their worth swallowed whole.

That's the war we fight. To stand proud beside our men, but never underneath them. To honor the culture while demanding our own damn space inside it.

An ol' lady isn't weak. She's steel wrapped in leather. She's a strategist, a mother, a keeper of secrets, and sometimes the only one keeping the chaos from collapsing into ruin.

And don't get it twisted; the patch may say "Property," but the spirit behind it is anything but owned.

They think submission means silence. Nah. In my world, submission means strength, choosing when I ride, and who's worth my fire. There was a time when being called someone's " ol' lady" would have made my skin crawl. But in the biker world, it's a title that's earned, not given. It means you're the one they trust, the ride-or-die, the backbone behind the patch. You're not invisible. You're respected. Revered. Maybe even feared. Because a real ol' lady knows how to hold it down and raise hell when necessary.

But let's get this straight, being an ol' lady never meant being owned. It means I walked into a world built by men and made a name without ever needing to raise my voice though sometimes, I did. I didn't come here to playhouse or be a wallflower. I came to build a life, raise a family, and still ride hard alongside my man.

If you're going to wear that title, wear it with pride. Not as property, but as power. Power to lead. Power to hold space. Power to show other women what self-respect looks like when you're covered in leather and loyalty.

But here's the truth they don't always tell you.

The "ol' lady rules" weren't written for women like me. I've watched too many women disappear behind someone else's patch. I've seen women lose themselves, their dreams, their self-worth. I wasn't passed around or patched over. Everything I learned in the clubhouse became the blueprint for what I promised my daughters I would never repeat.

What I Refuse to Pass Down

Here's what I won't leave to my daughters. I won't pass down silence. I won't pass down shame.

They will inherit my strength, not my trauma. They will learn that being loud doesn't mean being disrespectful. They will learn that boundaries are not walls. They are gates that swing open for the worthy.

Being a woman in this world means constantly navigating double standards, judgments, and invisible expectations. But I'll be damned if my daughters have to carry the same burdens I had to fight to put down.

So I teach them that their worth isn't up for debate. That shame is a lie people tell you when they fear your truth. That softness and strength are sisters, not opposites.

And when they look back at who raised them, I want them to see a woman who never played small to make others comfortable.

Breaking the Cycle

I learned how to survive by watching women around me fold. They folded to keep the peace. They folded to keep their man. They folded because they were never told they had another option.

My girls won't need permission to be powerful. I remember when my daughter wanted to wear her leather vest to school. She asked, 'Do I need permission?' I laughed and told her, 'Baby, the only permission you need is from yourself.' That's legacy.

That was the day I realized my fight wasn't just mine, it was hers, too. She put her vest on with pride.

What I want to hand my daughters isn't trauma wrapped in tradition.

I want to give them grace and grounded strength. At her first rally, my daughter froze when a group of men crowded too close. I leaned down and said, 'Stand tall. Look 'em in the eye. Don't flinch.' She did. That moment wasn't about toughness, it was about teaching her that grace and pride can ride side by side.

I want them to walk into any room, or rally, knowing they don't owe anyone an explanation for their worth.

In a world where motorcycle clubs hold strong values and rules, there's a woman who embodies the spirit of loyalty and honor. She faces many challenges and surprises that often leave people in shock. As she navigates through life, her experiences reveal deep confessions about what it means to be devoted.

Even when times get tough, she thrives on the support of her fellow club members, known as "Ol' Ladies." Together, they keep their code alive, sharing heartwarming stories along the way. The news spreads quickly among them, creating a community bound by respect and tradition.

I want my girls to say no, without apology.

To cry, without shame.

To fight for their own joy, on their own terms.

Because I've lived in survival mode. I've been the girl with street smarts, navigating broken systems and emotional landmines with no damn manual. And I became the woman who could raise daughters who aren't afraid to be whole.

In club life, traditional roles are often praised, he rides, she supports. But where is the line between respect and submission? Between being "his ol' lady" and being your own damn woman?

Respect in this world is currency. But so is power, and too often, women are expected to earn both by being quiet, loyal, and beautiful.

Let's challenge that.

I've learned that power doesn't always roar. Sometimes it whispers, "No." Sometimes it walks away. Sometimes it builds its own table, no permission.

You can be fierce. Feminine. Faithful.

To your club, to your man, and to yourself.

This isn't about throwing away tradition. It's about rewriting the fine print, so it includes women who ride their own path, with pride, with voice, and with strength.

"I respect the patch. But I never forget, I earned mine with fire, not silence."

We didn't sit at the head of the table, we built the table, fed it, and held it steady when the storm hit.
Because behind every patch and every man riding proud, there's a woman carrying fire and whether anyone admits it or not, the road runs straighter because of her.

The Women Beside the Patch

You want to understand club life? Then you'd better understand the women in it.

Now right around when I was 12 or 13 years old, I can tell a bit of a different story. The world was so different. I was thirteen when I watched an ol' lady shut down a drunk biker twice her size. She didn't scream. She didn't cry. She just planted her boots, stared him down, and said, 'Not today.' That was the first time I realized women weren't just accessories in this world, they were powerful.

Women have always stirred the pot in the biker scene. From riding their own bikes to sporting "property of" patches, we've been a hot topic for decades. But now? We're done being quiet. We're loud, proud, and taking up space.

Now, before I dive deeper into my thoughts on women in biking, let's set the stage. I rolled into this world back when women were pretty much put in a corner, seen but not heard.

And yeah, many bikers accepted that status quo. Why? Because their presence shook things up, especially within motorcycle clubs. Believe it or not, wars between major 1% clubs have kicked off over a woman! It sounds wild, but it's true.

So here I am, unapologetic and ready to share some truths about the challenges we face as women in this scene. Forget the myths; let's talk about reality, the heartwarming moments, the shocking confessions, and the rules we navigate every day.

Women like us are devoted riders who thrive against all odds, and trust me, our stories deserve to be told. Not the ones you see in crime shows getting tossed between scenes like props. Not the ones half-naked on Instagram pretending to know what riding two-up even means. I'm talking about the real ones.

The ones who ride. The ones who serve. The ones who lead. The ones who hold it down when everything's burning around them. The women beside the patch.

Ol' lady Isn't an Insult

Some women in this life put the guys to shame. In outlaw biker clubs, we ride hard and love harder. This isn't about just rocking a patch, it's about living a code that most people couldn't handle for five minutes.

Like the night I sat in an ER waiting room, blood on my boots, still clutching a brother's cut. Nurses whispered, people stared, but I didn't care. I was there to hold the line until he came out breathing. That's what loyalty looks like. He was stabbed in a bar fight and I stayed with him all night.

Let's get real, these clubs draw us in with their dangerous allure. The thrill of being part of something notorious electrifies our veins, giving us that adrenaline rush that makes life worth living. We thrive on respect, sure, but let's be honest, sometimes it's all about the fear we strike into outsiders' hearts too.

I've seen some shocking stuff along the way, faced with challenges that would make most people falter, yet here I am, unapologetically devoted to my sisters and brothers.

Let's get this clear, " ol' lady" is not a slur. It's not some caveman term for ownership. In the right club, with the right man, it's a title earned with patience, and unwavering loyalty.

Being an ol' lady means you hold rank, not on paper, maybe, but in reality.

You know the schedule and you hold onto the secrets tightly. Your job is to clean up messes and mend bruises while keeping chaos at bay.

You manage all this with style, eyeliner on point and steel-toe boots laced up. If you like me you are always ready for the worse and hope for the best.

In the world of motorcycle clubs, being a woman isn't easy. There are rules to follow and an honor code to uphold.

As an ol' lady, you face huge challenges every day. But even through shocking confessions and forgotten moments, your devotion shines brightly. You thrive in this wildlife, navigating the stops and drives that come your way. And when big news hits, it's your values that guide you, heartwarming as ever.

I remember a time when the club was under intense scrutiny. It felt like we were constantly being watched, every move dissected. During one such tense day, I was at the club's bar, trying to keep spirits high. I noticed a new face. A young woman, clearly overwhelmed by the atmosphere. She reminded me of myself when I first entered this world, unsure but eager to belong.

I approached her, offering a joke and a drink. We talked for hours, sharing stories and laughter, her apprehension slowly dissolving. It was in that moment I realized the power we hold as ol' ladies. Not just in handling chaos but in nurturing new bonds, creating a sense of home amid the chaos. That day, I wasn't just a protector of secrets; I became a mentor, a guide, passing down the wisdom of resilience and loyalty that defines us.

Years later, the club evolved. The once unsure young woman had become a formidable leader. Watching her, it was clear she had become a beacon of hope, not just for the club, but the entire neighborhood. Her initiative blossomed into a movement, drawing diverse people to our cause.

At the event's end, she approached me, fulfilled. "We've come so far," she said. I nodded, proud. "And it's just the beginning," I replied.

We knew we had created something special, a testament to transformation, shared vision, and community strength.

I've been an ol' lady long enough to know it's not for the weak.

It's for the wise.

Patchless Power

Some of the most powerful women I know never wore a cut. They led from the edges. They kept the club alive when the men were too broken or too blind to see the bigger picture.

I've held men together in hospital waiting rooms, fed 50 people with donated groceries, cleaned up messes no one admits they made, and supported women whose husbands never came home.

I've seen sisters pull me out of hell when I stayed too long. I've done the same for them.

Sisterhood isn't soft here.
It's steel.

These ol' ladies, make the calls no one else wants to make. And they do it all with no title, just heart. I've seen tough tattooed women that are wild-hearted hold a brotherhood together while holding babies and burying brothers in the same weekend.

The Line Between Respect and Submission

Too often, women are told to earn both by being quiet, loyal, and pretty.

I don't buy that. Power doesn't always roar. Sometimes it whispers no. Sometimes it walks away. Sometimes it builds its own table, no permission.

And one bad apple can rot a lot of good fruit.

Some of us don't ride behind a man. We ride beside him. Or ahead of him. Always on our own if we can.

I ride my own. There's nothing like gripping your own handlebars, knowing the road answers to you. There's something spiritual about grabbing the throttle and letting the road remind you who the hell you are.

More and more women are doing it now, owning Harleys, joining *all-female clubs*, and showing up at rallies with just as much thunder as the guys.

More women are riding than ever in clubs, solo, loud and proud. We're not going anywhere.

Femininity is not an apology. It's strategy.

I can be loud, wild, and strong as hell, and still wear lashes and lipstick to a rally. I can pitch a tent, roll with the boys, curse like a sailor, and still demand dignity.

Femininity is power. It's strategy. It's mine.

We ride the line between boldness and boundaries. We call out bullshit. We roll on. It's strategy. It's power. It's ours. I'll tell you straight: being an Ole Lady isn't for the faint of heart. We ride a thin line between loyalty and self-respect, and let's be real, people love to toss around their stereotypes about outlaw biker women like they're candy at a parade. News flash: we aren't just pretty faces in leather vests; we're fierce, resilient forces with our own lives and stories.

Sure, the world expects us to play nice, keep our mouths shut, and grin through all that sexist nonsense. But I won't sugarcoat it, I've had enough of those outdated expectations.

Our rules? Respect your patch holders in public, stay sharp as the club's eyes and ears, and know when to speak up or stay quiet. It's all part of our code of honor.

Don't get me wrong; there are challenges everywhere. We face them head-on, showing strength where others see weakness. And while we support our men and the club, that doesn't mean we forget who we are or what we want. Each time we ride out, we leave behind judgments and embrace our power, not just as bikers but as women on our terms.

Sisterhood, Not Scraps

We need each other, ladies.

This lifestyle can chew you up if you don't have a circle of women who understand. I've had biker sisters wipe my tears, stitch my leather, hide my secrets, and drag my ass out of situations I had no business surviving. And I've done the same for them.

It isn't always pretty. But it's real.

One night, I swung a little too hard in a fight, and before I knew it, my sister grabbed my belt loop, yanked me back, and said, 'Not today, babe.' We laughed all the way home. That memory says more about sisterhood than any speech ever could.

And if you're a woman reading this, whether you ride, support, or serve, there's room for you here. But only if you're willing to honor the road, the code, and the women who paved it before you.

In the world of biker women, it's easy to get tangled up in

what we think loyalty means. We often wear our patches like armor, believing they define us and bind us to certain rules, rules that are sometimes steeped more in fear than love. So, let's break this down, no BS.

Love or Fear—Check Your Engine

Love will make you show up because you choose to. Fear will make you perform so you don't get left behind. I've ridden for both and I've paid for both. Loyalty, like love, is only holy when it's free.

Love is fierce; it gives you courage when the odds are stacked against you. It's that electric feeling when you're cruising down an open road, wind whipping through your hair, knowing you've got a tribe who has your back. That's where true loyalty lies, when you choose to be there for each other simply because you care.

Now, flip the coin over to fear. Fear can twist loyalty into something heavy and burdensome. Are you showing up at club events or holding onto those patch rules because you genuinely believe in them? Or is it because you're scared of being abandoned, judged, or left behind?

Love can anchor you or chain you. In my world, loyalty was currency and sometimes love cost more than it gave back.

The next thing you need to understand is simple;
Behind every act of loyalty is a wound that taught it.

And those wounds?

They tell their own stories.

Chapter 6 Legacy Reflection Questions

1. What role have women played in shaping your strength, identity, or sense of community?

2. Have you ever confused femininity with weakness, either in yourself or someone else? What shifted that belief?

3. How can you better support or uplift the women riding beside you, in any area of your life?

CHAPTER 7: HEARTSTRINGS, HEARTACHES & DEVOTION

"Trust isn't given; it's earned in sweat, silence, and storm."

It's everywhere, stitched onto patches, inked into skin, and boomed from mouths that wouldn't survive a loyalty test in a hurricane, let alone a biker bar. Seriously, what happened to honor? Did it get lost between the handlebars and the last cold beer?

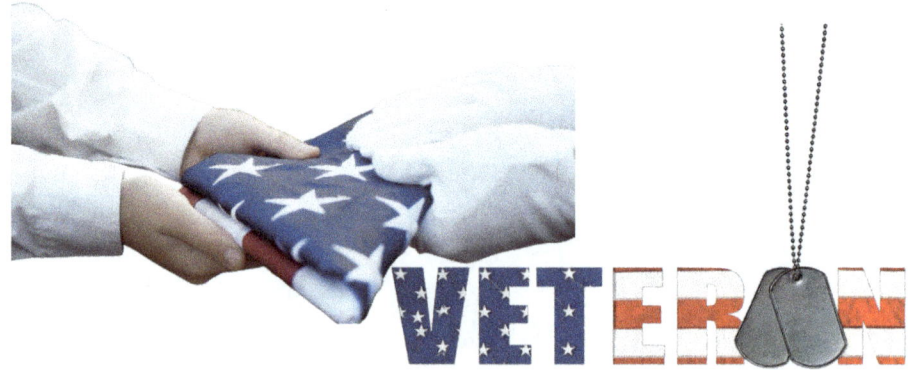

"Some oaths save you. Some slice you open."
People talk about loyalty like it's cardboard, flat, simple, one-sided.
In the biker world? Loyalty is a damn blade.
It'll protect you... or cut you clean through.
I learned early that loyalty isn't proven in big moments, loud rooms, or dramatic speeches. It's proven in silence.

In who shows up when no one's watching. In who stands still when the storm hits instead of sprinting for the exit. And trust me, I've weathered enough storms to know the difference.

My whole life, I've been "claimed" by people who loved the idea of me the strong one, the fighter, the dependable one, the woman who keeps going even when the world is trying to bury her.

Being the strong one is great... until one day you break, and everyone looks confused, like,

"Wait... YOU? You're not allowed to fall apart."

Meanwhile the people who carried me through hell?

Most didn't share blood with me.

Some didn't even share my last name.

But they shared backbone and that's thicker than DNA.

The Night I learned Who My Real People Were

There was a night when everything in my life felt like it was unraveling my body was flaring, my marriage was crumbling, my identity felt like it was slipping through my fingers.

I was exhausted, in pain, and too damn tired to pretend I was okay. I called someone I thought would be there for me.

They didn't answer.

I texted.

Nothing.

Meanwhile, one of my biker sisters, someone who didn't "owe" me a thing, showed up at my house with a cup of gas-station coffee, a hoodie, and that look that said:

"Say the word and we ride."

No judgment.

No questions.

Just presence.

That's loyalty.

Not who says they love you but who puts boots on the ground when you're too broken to stand.

In that moment, I realized the true meaning of friendship. It wasn't about grand gestures or constant communication; it was about being there when it truly mattered, in the quiet moments of despair and uncertainty. My biker sister's silent support spoke volumes more than any words of comfort could.

We sat together. It was exactly what I needed, a reminder that I wasn't alone, even when it felt like the world was crumbling around me.

As we sipped our Surside's and watched the sun dip below the horizon, I felt a renewed sense of strength. With her by my side, I knew I could face whatever came next. Together, we were unstoppable, ready to take on the world. Tomorrow!

The Lies We Tell Ourselves About Loyalty

Let's get honest.

Most of us learned loyalty the wrong damn way:
- Loyalty means staying quiet.
- Loyalty means staying small.
- Loyalty means tolerating disrespect.
- Loyalty means pretending everything is fine.

Wrong.

Loyalty that requires you to disappear is not loyalty.

It's hostage-taking.

And I refused to keep being held hostage.

As the last sliver of sun dipped below the horizon, I turned to her, ready to share my epiphany. "You know," I started, my voice steady like the tide, "we've been fed some real tall tales about loyalty, haven't we?"

She nodded, a knowing smile playing at her lips. "Yeah, we have. But it's time we rewrite those stories."

The Man Who Proved What Loyalty Wasn't

I once loved a man who talked a good game. He was loud, charming, always the center of the crowd. He told everyone he was loyal. Like it was his whole personality.

But when life threw a punch?

He folded like wet cardboard.

One night, after a scare that sent me back to the hospital, I came home weak, shaking, terrified of what the test results might say.

I expected him to sit with me.

Hold my hand.

Say nothing, just be there.

Instead?

He went out drinking with the boys because he "needed to clear his head."

I learned something that night!

Some men want the story of a strong woman. But they don't want the work of standing beside one.

Meanwhile, a biker brother I barely knew at the time dropped off soup on my porch.

Didn't knock. Didn't make it about him.

Just left the care package without the performance.

That is loyalty.

Quiet.

Steady.

Un-spectacular.

Real.

When Loyalty Is A Lesson – Not a Lifestyle

Here's the thing, you can be loyal without being stupid. Once I stopped bending over backwards for people who wouldn't lift a finger for me, my life changed.

My circle shrank and thank God it did.

The people who remained?
- They don't flinch when I'm sick.
- They don't disappear when I'm loud.
- They don't judge the patches on my back or the scars on my body.
- They don't expect perfection — just honesty.

That's the loyalty I want my kids to see. Not the kind that keeps you trapped, but the kind that builds you back.

It's the kind of loyalty that encourages growth, understanding, and mutual respect. It teaches them that real relationships are not transactional but built on genuine care and support. As they navigate their own paths, I hope they learn to recognize the difference between those who are truly there for them and those who only appear during convenient times.

I want them to know that it's okay to let go of relationships that drain them, to embrace those who uplift them, and to never compromise their self-worth for the sake of someone else's comfort. True loyalty doesn't demand you to lose yourself; instead, it celebrates who you are and who you are becoming.

This is the lesson I hope to pass on. That loyalty should be a source of strength, a bond that enriches your life, and a foundation upon which you can build your dreams.

Humor Break - The Reality of Biker "Loyalty"

Let me tell you something funny;

People assume biker loyalty means every man in a vest is automatically reliable.

Ha.
Hahaha.
Heh.

Look, I love my brothers.

But if you want to know the truth?

Some of them are loyal as hell.

Some can't even be loyal to their own motorcycles.
If a man has three bikes and all of them are broken, don't expect him to be emotionally available.

And loyalty in a clubhouse?

It's like finding matching socks in a biker's laundry basket, possible... but rare.

But when it's real?

It's unbeatable.

We Raise Leaders, Not Just Riders

Some of us are raising college kids, and don't you dare act surprised.

I've seen biker families grind to give their kids a better shot. I've watched patches throw together scholarships and fundraisers to send young women to med school and keep sons off the streets.

Some of those "rough-looking dudes" you see outside the clubhouse?

They're damn proud daddies who show up to every graduation in boots and shades, with tears in their eyes and pride in their chest. They're the proudest of fathers, behind those rugged exteriors lie hearts full of love and commitment.

We may ride hard, but we raise harder.

The Price of Being Loyal To Yourself

This part is the hardest to swallow.

Sometimes, the person you betray most...is yourself.

I betrayed myself every time I stayed silent to keep peace.

Every time I carried weight no one else offered to share.

Every time I gave loyalty to people who only gave me excuses.

Illness forced me to learn self-loyalty.

Biker life sharpened it.

Your body can betray you.

People can betray you.

But your choices?

That's your territory.

Your power.

Your final line in the sand.

And once you realize that, everything changes. You start to recognize the importance of your own voice and the weight of your own decisions. You understand that setting boundaries is not just about keeping others out, but about keeping yourself intact.

Self-loyalty becomes a daily practice. A commitment to honor your own needs and desires, to speak your truth even when it shakes the ground beneath you. It's about standing firm in your choices, knowing that they define who you are, not just to the world, but to yourself.

In the clubhouse, loyalty can be a currency, traded and bartered, sometimes lost in the noise of revving engines and the chaos of the road. But the loyalty you hold for yourself? That's the quiet strength that keeps you riding, no matter the terrain. It's the compass that guides you home, back to a place where you are truly at peace with who you are.

Because loyalty isn't just a club rule or a relationship expectation it's the foundation of every community you belong to.

And in the biker world?
Community isn't a concept.
It's action.
Especially when someone needs help.

Which leads to the truth I learned next:

Not all loyalty looks like brotherhood. Sometimes the strongest loyalty comes from the women — the ones who hold the world together when the men are too busy blowing it apart.

Chapter 7 Legacy Reflection Questions

1. Who has earned your loyalty, and who has only borrowed it?

2. Where have you stayed loyal at the cost of your own peace?

3. Who showed up for you when life got quiet, painful, or ugly — and what did that teach you?

4. How can you practice loyalty to yourself first, without apology?

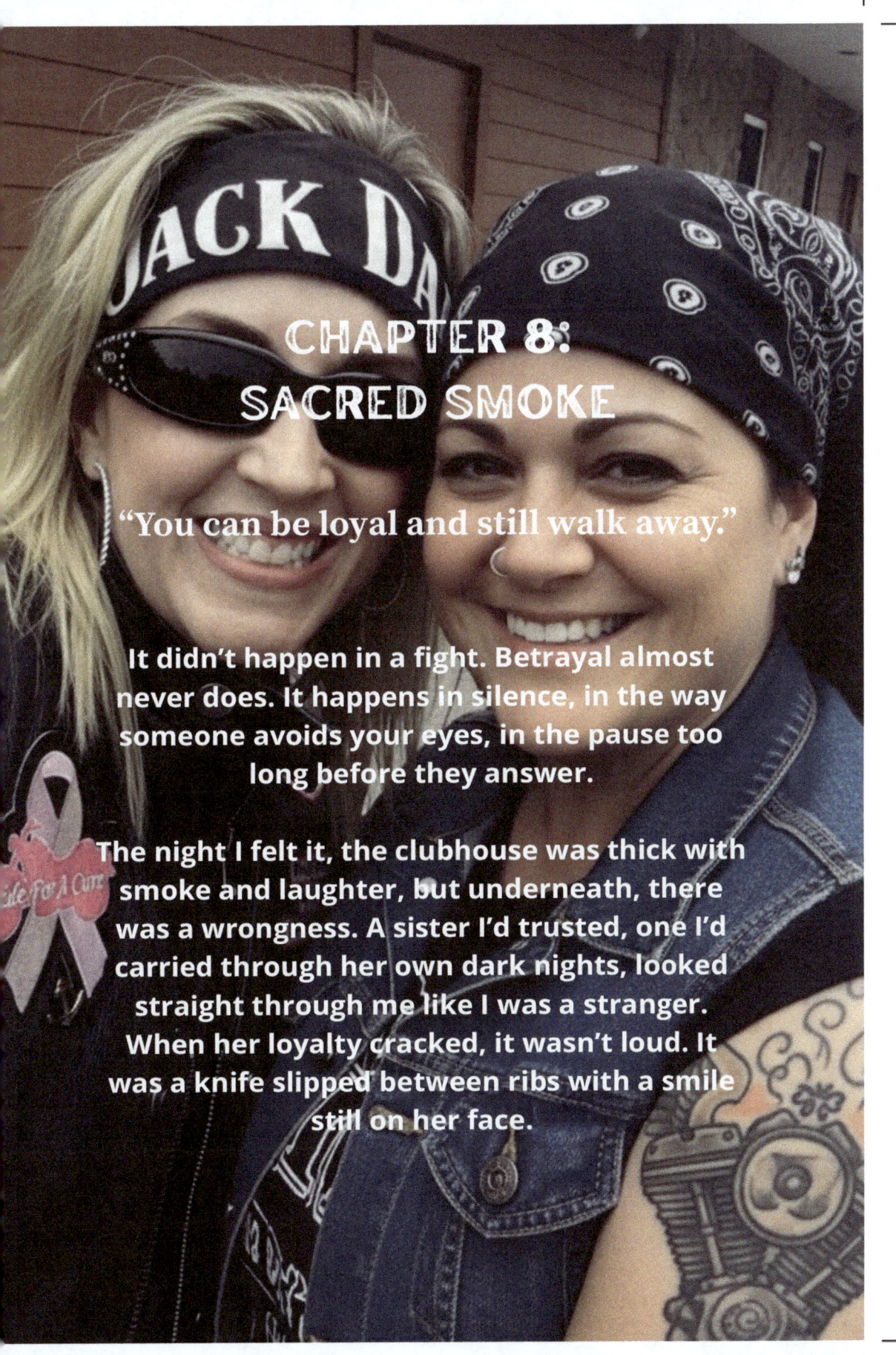

CHAPTER 8:
SACRED SMOKE

"You can be loyal and still walk away."

It didn't happen in a fight. Betrayal almost never does. It happens in silence, in the way someone avoids your eyes, in the pause too long before they answer.

The night I felt it, the clubhouse was thick with smoke and laughter, but underneath, there was a wrongness. A sister I'd trusted, one I'd carried through her own dark nights, looked straight through me like I was a stranger. When her loyalty cracked, it wasn't loud. It was a knife slipped between ribs with a smile still on her face.

No gunfire. No brawl. Just the hollow sound of something breaking inside me. That's the truth they don't tell you. Fists heal faster than broken bonds. However, many of you have felt that in your life at some point.

I walked out into the night, leather heavy on my shoulders, air colder than it should've been. That was the moment I learned betrayal doesn't bleed you on the outside. It stains the soul. And you never really wash it out.

More Than the Mayhem

You won't see this on the news. You'll see mugshots, yes. You'll see raids and crime charts and drug busts with leather jackets piled in the evidence room. But what you won't see, what they never show, is the line of bikes stretching two miles deep for a child with leukemia.

You won't see the club that just covered the funeral costs for a young widow left with nothing but memories and heartache. No cameras rolling. No hashtags trending just real people stepping up when it counts. Because here's the kicker, behind those tough exteriors and loud engines lies a heart bigger than most would ever guess.

The media loves to paint broad strokes. Casting shadows over anyone who rides with patches on their backs. But if you look closer. You'll find stories of kindness buried beneath the headlines.

So next time you catch a glimpse of those mugshots flashing across your screen, remember not all heroes wear capes.

Some ride motorcycles and they don't need the limelight to do good.

Because that kind of story?

Doesn't sell papers, or news. You don't hear people telling stories about stained souls.

But it's real. And it happens all the time.

Take, for instance, a young boy we know named Mason. We organized a summer ride for him. At just eight years old, bald from chemotherapy, he stood in the parking lot alongside his mother. I'll never forget how small he appeared in the oversized helmet we provided, clutching his stuffed bear in one hand while the other reached out to touch the chrome of a Harley like it was magic.

Hundreds of us rolled in, engines echoing like thunder, and when we cut the bikes, you could hear him laughing from across the lot. He rode shotgun with the president that day, grinning so wide it felt like the sun cracked through the clouds just for him. His mom cried the whole time, not because she was sad, but because for those few hours, her kid wasn't a cancer patient. He was a warrior with an army at his back. He was one of many that got to ride that day.

You won't see that on CNN.

You also won't see the patched man delivering groceries to an old widow on his own dime. You won't see the crew repainting a homeless vet's house on a Sunday morning after riding all night.

Behind Every Clubhouse Door

Walk into a clubhouse and you might find a loud bar, some

patched-up men, and a cloud of cigar smoke. But keep looking.
Look past the leather.
Look past the attitude.

You'll see donation jars. Signup sheets. Wall photos of fundraisers, memorial runs, and rally awards for "Most Funds Raised." You'll see women organizing spaghetti dinners for multiple events. You'll see veterans who found family again. You'll see men crying over the loss of a brother, then turning that pain into action.

Stick around long enough and you'll see a tribe with a mission.

Why We Show Up

Bikers know pain. We've lost friends and buried brothers. We've faced the edge of self-destruction more times than we can count. Every scar is a reminder of the values that hold us together.

So when someone else is hurting? We feel it in our bones, down to our souls.

We don't need a nonprofit tax form to step up. We don't need approval from city council to serve. We show up because we know what it means to feel abandoned. And when we ride? We ride loud enough to make sure no one feels alone.

There was the time the Pagan chapter rallied together and raised over $20,000 for a child fighting cancer. No one asked for credit. No one did it for the headlines. They did it because that's what family does—ride out for the ones who can't fight alone.

Then there was the all-women's crew, fierce and unstoppable, who organized a suicide awareness ride. Five hundred bikes thundered down the highway, each one a testament to survival, sisterhood, and the kind of love that refuses to let anyone go quietly. The roar of engines was more than noise. It was a promise, you're not alone.

In the Northeast, clubs banded together for a Christmas ride. They loaded up bikes with gifts and delivered them to over a thousand children in shelters. For some kids, it was the only holiday magic they'd see all year. For the riders, it was a reminder that giving back is the real badge of honor.

And when COVID hit, MCs didn't just hunker down. They ran supply routes, delivering food and medicine to high-risk elders in rural towns, places most people forget exist. No one wore capes, but plenty wore leather and grit.

Not all clubs are saints. Some are messy, loud, and imperfect. But many are warrior-hearted. They show up, boots on the ground, when the world needs more than words. That's the kind of loyalty I believe in. The kind that rides out for strangers, stands up for the vulnerable, and proves that family is built on backbone, not just blood.

A Different Kind of Brotherhood

Some people build legacy through wealth. We build it through service.

You might not see our names on plaques. You might not read about us in history books. But when shit goes down in a community? We're the ones showing up. Sometimes

before the sirens. Sometimes after the cameras leave.
We're not perfect. But we're present. And that's more than most people can say.

Don't Call It PR

Some folks say clubs only do charity to look good. Here's my response: I watched an entire club mobilize like an army. Within a week, they raised twenty grand. Within a month, the clubhouse walls were covered in thank-you cards from strangers who'd never met a person but felt the roar of a community behind them.

That's the good they don't talk about.

They don't show the patched man dropping off groceries at an old woman's porch.

They don't show the women organizing toy runs that put Christmas under trees for kids with nothing.

They don't show the veterans finding a family again, long after the military cut them loose.

Why? Because kindness doesn't sell. Blood does.

And in the end, isn't that what truly matters? The unseen ripples of kindness, spreading quietly but surely, making the world a better place one act at a time.

The reality is that the stories worth telling are often the ones that go unnoticed, whispered in the quiet corners of life, where true impact is made not for applause, but for the sheer joy of giving. It's about the silent heroes who expect nothing in return, those who find their riches not in wealth, but in the smiles and gratitude they inspire.

But make no mistake, there's more heart behind those vests than most churches can fit in their pews.

We don't ride just for rebellion. We ride for remembrance, for rescue, for recovery. We ride because we know what it feels like to be abandoned, and we refuse to let anyone else feel that way if we can stop it.

We do it when no one's watching. We ride 150 miles for a cause no one's heard of and we donate anonymously to people who will never know our names.

Because it's not about image. It's about impact.

If we wanted attention, we'd post selfies with our lattes and call it a day. But this life isn't about likes. It's about legacies. Because the best recognition doesn't come with a spotlight or a plaque. It's like being a ninja in a world full of show-offs, quiet but impactful. And why do we help people who will never know our names? Because at the end of the day, it's not about us. It's about making a difference, even if it means being just another ghost in the machine. So go ahead, keep saying charities are all about appearances. We'll be here proving you wrong, one humble act at a time.

When I think about the people I love, it hits me hard where I've fallen short in sharing their full truth. It's easy to get caught up in the good stuff, the laughter, the victories, and those badass moments that make us feel invincible. But let's not sugarcoat things or wear blinders like some cliché biker chick trying to fit into a mold.

Let's get real people are like onions. Or better yet, motorcycles, beautiful, badass machines with a whole lot of parts that sometimes bang into each other like the drummer in a biker band who can't quite keep the beat. I've gotta admit, there've been plenty of times I've glossed over the rusty bits, choosing instead to shine up the chrome and make everyone look like a gleaming Harley on a Sunday ride.

Where did I mess up? Probably when I turned my favorite characters into superhero cartoons, ignoring the fact that even heroes have bad hair days and fender benders. Or maybe I slapped on a fresh coat of paint over their flaws because the truth was a little too gritty, like a chain that needs tightening.

Life's got the whole kit and caboodle, the good, the bad, and whatever the hell else's rattling around in the engine. Sure, we're tough as nails with leather jackets and steel nerves, but that doesn't mean we can't own up when we're scared, lost, or just plain confused. Those moments? They rev our engines just as much as the wins.

So, let's crank the throttle on honesty, put our voices in gear, and tell the stories of the people we love, the whole, messy, beautiful ride.

The worst wounds don't bleed. They walk around with your memories, smiling like nothing ever broke.
So next time you see a line of bikes stretching two miles deep, know this: they're not just riding for noise. They're riding for someone's life.

But faith and ritual don't shield you from betrayal. Sometimes the knives come not from enemies, but from the very brothers and sisters you trusted most.

Chapter 8 Legacy Reflection Questions

1. Have you ever been surprised by kindness from an unexpected source? What did it teach you?

2. How do you define service or giving back? Is it tied to visibility, or something deeper?

3. In your own life, where can you show up more for others without expecting recognition?

CHAPTER 9:
KNIVES BEHIND THE PATCH THE BIKER CODE & THE FEMINIST FIGHT

"You can live by the code and still rewrite the rules."

The first time I watched Sons of Anarchy, I laughed so hard I nearly choked on my drink. Not because it was funny, but because it was a circus dressed up as a mirror.
There they were, men brooding under perfect lighting, women reduced to background noise, plot twists about drugs and guns like they were gospel truth. Anyone who's lived this life could spot the bullshit from a mile away.

I remember pausing mid-episode, looking around my living room, and thinking,
If this is what people believe about us, no wonder the world gets it so wrong.

Because the truth is, most clubs aren't crime dramas on two wheels. They're families. They're flawed, messy, loud, loyal, heartbreaking families.

And women? We're not just props. We're the backbone. We keep the engines running when the men can't. We hold the weight no patch ever could.

Hollywood glamorizes the chaos, but it never shows the aftermath. The empty boots at the funeral. The women scraping together rent while their men rot in jail. The wives juggling three jobs, the mothers soothing kids who heard too much whispered about their fathers.

SOA gave the world a fantasy.
My life gave me scars.

When Clubs Become Community, Not Chaos

Here's the part they'll never film, the compassion. The brotherhood that shows up before the cops, the fundraisers that bury children with dignity, the quiet loyalty that doesn't need a soundtrack to matter.

Real clubs run fundraisers, deliver food, support veterans, move mountains quietly because it's the right thing to do, not because there's a camera rolling.

Some clubs have redefined what it means to wear a patch.

These aren't just riding crews. They're community builders. Mentors. Movement-makers. They saw the need for more than fast bikes and fierce loyalty, and they stepped up.

Take, for instance, the Iron Guardians. Sure, they can tear up a highway faster than you can say "road trip," but when they're not busy eating asphalt, they're organizing food drives that put most grocery stores to shame. Last year alone, they collected enough canned goods to feed an entire zip code.

And still looked cool doing it.

Then there's the Steel Stallions, who traded in their wild rides for community outreach programs. They've teamed up with local schools to teach kids about bike safety, and let's be real, if anyone knows how to avoid wipeout, it's these seasoned riders.

Their motto?
"Teach them young, so they don't end up like us."

It's both hilarious and heartwarming. Half joke, half truth.

These aren't gangs.
They're guardians.
They protect their neighborhoods.
They show up for strangers.
They hold their communities together with raw heart and stubborn loyalty.

And me?
I've handed out toys in December when my own joints were

screaming.
I've packed meals with bikers who barely had money themselves.
I've stood shoulder to shoulder with men and women who knew pain intimately and still chose service.

They don't teach you this in law school.
But it saves lives.

From Rebels to Resources

In a world where community support feels like a fossil, some clubs said,
 "Screw waiting , we'll do it ourselves."

I've watched clubs turn garages into emergency shelters faster than FEMA turns on a microphone.

Some clubs have created entire community programs, offering food, shelter, and support for families in need. Others run veteran support rides, suicide prevention campaigns, or school supply drives that rival what your local government does.

I've seen:
- **Highway adoption crews** cleaning the same stretches of road every month
- **Veteran support convoys** rolling through towns louder than any parade
- **Suicide prevention rides** raising awareness without shame
- **School supply drives** that put city programs to shame
- **Fundraisers for assault and trafficking survivors** hosted with more dignity than half the "official" orgs do

Clubs like these don't just ride — they rebuild.

And for the record, some of the most powerful people in a club don't wear patches.

They're the women in jeans, ponytails, and steel-toe boots running the raffle tables, organizing the routes, feeding the riders, and keeping the ecosystem alive.

In a world where community support often feels like a distant memory, some clubs are stepping up to the plate like it's their last chance at bat. Forget waiting for local governments to act, these grassroots heroes are rolling up their sleeves and getting to work.

It's the kind of quiet leadership the world dismisses until it collapses without us.

Loyalty, Womanhood, and the Feminist Fight

Let's talk about the code and where it collides with being a woman who refuses to shrink.

Loyalty isn't submission.
(And trust me, submission is only used in ONE room of the house and it ain't the clubhouse.)

Loyalty is choice.
Loyalty is fire.
Loyalty is standing beside your people without losing yourself in the process.

The real feminist fight in biker culture isn't about overthrowing men — it's about refusing to be erased.

It's knowing when to call out bullshit and when to keep your powder dry.

It's riding your own bike, or riding behind someone you trust without apology for either.

It's claiming space the old way by walking in like you own your story.

I've seen women lead rides, run chapters, raise money, and hold the emotional line better than half the men wearing patches.

I've also seen the other side the women who weaponize loyalty, chase patches, stir chaos, and drag everyone down with them.

Not all women in this life are the same.
And thank God for that, because the ones who show up with real heart? They're the steel that holds the brotherhood, the community, and the culture together.

When Loyalty Cuts Both Ways

Loyalty is beautiful until it isn't. And here's the part few outsiders understand. Most wounds in biker life don't come from enemies. They come from people at your own table. Not every betrayal has a gun involved.

Sometimes it's a whisper.
A lie.
A secret.
A trust broken so cleanly it feels surgical.
The world doesn't see that part.
They think chaos comes from the outside.
But you and I both know, **the deepest knives are carried behind the patch.**

In this world of deep connections and even deeper betrayals, the most painful wounds often come from those who once shared your laughter and dreams. Loyalty here is a delicate dance, requiring a balance between faith and vigilance. It's about knowing when to stand firm and when to walk away, even if it means leaving behind what you thought was unbreakable.

I remember a time when I thought I had found my tribe, a group that understood me like no other. We rode together, shared personal stories around bar tables, and built dreams events we attended. There was a particular friend, someone I considered a sister, who was always by my side. We laughed together, cried together, and supported each other through thick and thin.

But the trust I placed in her was not as unshakeable as I believed. One day, I discovered she had been spreading lies about me, turning others in the group against me. It was a betrayal that cut deeper than any outsider could. The pain was immense, not just because of the deceit, but because it came from someone I thought would always have my back.

Amidst the shadows of betrayal, there's an undeniable light in the camaraderie that transcends bloodlines, in shared journeys that forge unyielding bonds. It's found in late-night rides, where silence speaks louder than words, and the sound of the engines becomes a shared heartbeat.

True loyalty, the kind that heals rather than cuts, is both rare and precious. It's seen in the eyes of a friend who stands by you when the road is rough, who celebrates your triumphs and mourns your losses as if they were their own.

For those who embrace this life sincerely, understanding that loyalty is both a gift and a responsibility, they find a family forged by choice, not blood. This family, with its flaws and glory, forms the heart of the brotherhood, the soul of the road, and the spirit of freedom that can never truly be tamed. Yet, betrayal lurks, a sharp knife wielded by those close, cutting deeper than any outsider ever could.

And that's why the next part of my story isn't about Hollywood versions of danger.

It's about the real kind.
The kind that shows up in courtrooms.

In informant files.
In the quiet moments when the people you'd die for prove they'd never do the same.

Because while illness taught me who I could trust...
club life taught me who I absolutely couldn't.

And once you learn that?

Nothing...
not the law, not the lies, not the patch.....
ever looks the same again.

Chapter 9 Legacy Reflection Questions

1. What's one cause or community effort you've seen a club support that changed your view of the lifestyle? Did it shift your perspective? Did it inspire you to get involved?

2. If you had your own patch or crew, what kind of "good trouble" would you raise hell for? Be specific. Think local. Think loud.

3. Who is someone in your life who leads quietly but powerfully, like the clubs that do the work with no applause? How do they influence your ride, your voice, your purpose?

4. What does leadership look like in your life? How are you using your voice or presence to make a difference?

5. Who in your world is "changing the game" quietly? How can you honor their work?

CHAPTER 10: FAMILY BY FIRE

"Power isn't loud. Sometimes, it's the choice to stay silent, or to speak when it burns."

Loss in this life doesn't wait for permission. It sneaks in between laughter and smoke, and suddenly the seat next to you is empty.

Illness showed me who would hold my hand through hell, but club life? That taught me who would sell me out for a cigarette and a story. One minute you're laughing with people you'd die for, and the next you're staring at paperwork in some office with your name written in someone else's handwriting.

Betrayal doesn't always come with a bang. Sometimes it arrives disguised as "brotherhood," handed over by the very person you thought would bleed before they ever broke your trust.

And maybe that's why Redman's funeral hit me the way it did. Because standing there, surrounded by hundreds of bikes glinting under a heavy gray sky, I was reminded what real loyalty actually looks like and how rare it is.
I'll never forget that day.

The church couldn't hold the crowd, so they moved the celebration to a huge property, big enough for the weight of his life and the people who loved him. Bikes lined the whole horizon, chrome catching the light like a thousand tiny goodbyes.

I stood by his pictures, leather warming on my shoulders, wishing he'd bust out of that urn one last time with that wild grin, telling us to quit crying and fire up the damn engines. So we did.

The rumble rolled across the field like thunder, a thousand heartbeats trying to fill the silence he left behind.

A band played while we ate what he would've called his "last feast." Stories poured out. The kind that make you laugh until you choke, then cry because you know you'll never hear them again from the man himself.

Netflix won't ever show this part of biker life.
No perfect lighting.
No dramatic music.
Just raw engines in the dark, each one a voice raised for someone who can't speak anymore.

Redman was the original biker Santa ! Collecting toys for tots, donations, laughter, and good karma everywhere he went.

A one-man charity machine with a heart bigger than his bike. And as the night settled and the engines cooled, I realized something hard and holy. Some people would never betray you. Some people earn their patch with their soul, not their signature.

Some people are proof that loyalty still exists even when others prove it doesn't.

And that's where this story turns.

From the people who loved me right...
to the ones who tried to burn me down.

The Business of Brotherhood

Let's talk real.

For some clubs, the line between brotherhood and business got blurred a long damn time ago.
And when loyalty turns into leverage?
When patches become products?
When the ride becomes a hustle?

Everything shifts.

Running a club ain't cheap. Anyone who's ever rebuilt a carburetor at 2 a.m. knows that. Bikes break down at the worst possible times (thanks for nothing, engineering gods). BBQs cost more than your rent. Lawyers? Yeah, they don't take hugs or favors. So fundraising matters. It always has.

But something changes when the mission stops being about the miles and starts being about the money.

There was a time we rode just to feel alive, open road, open throttle, no spreadsheets, no budgets, no "projected revenue" for next month's rally. Now you're standing around a table arguing over how many shirts need sold before the next patch order can go in. And don't even get me started on sponsorships.

In the beginning, a patch meant loyalty. It meant you were all in, heart, grit, and brotherhood.

But somewhere along the line, that same patch started looking like a damn logo to the outside world. A logo corporations thought they could buy, brand, or use however they wanted.

Here's the truth nobody likes to admit.
The moment you let someone slap their name across your leather?
You're not a biker anymore.
You're an unpaid billboard with a heartbeat.

Sure, the perks look shiny. Free gear, "VIP" invites, discounts at bars where the floor sticks to your boots. But those perks come with strings. And those strings get pulled real quick.

One demand letter in your mailbox and suddenly you're

learning more trademark law than any biker should ever need to know.

And that's the slippery slope.

It starts with a fundraiser, a genuine one. To bury a brother or help a family. Nothing wrong with that. That's the heart of the culture. But give it a few years and suddenly every damn weekend is an event, a charity ride, a merch table, a negotiation. Brotherhood becomes branding.

Some clubs have traded their heart for hustle.

Their legacy for liability.

Their loyalty for "like and subscribe."

What started as camaraderie becomes commerce.

And that's where the cracks start forming. The same cracks that betrayal slides right through.

Not Every Club Sells Out

Let's get something straight before anyone twists my words: not every motorcycle club has lost its damn soul.

There are still clubs out there that run like old-school family kitchens. They are warm, tight, and have no room for egos, but always room for one more plate. The kind of clubs where loyalty isn't bought with merch or measured in event profits.

Where decisions still get made the way they were always meant to.

✓ church meetings
✓ votes that mean something
✓ voices that matter
✓ brotherhood over business

They're rare now.
That's why they matter.

Hollywood doesn't show these clubs. Too boring, not enough gunfire or exploding gas stations. But the truth? These clubs are the heartbeat of MC culture. The ones who kept the roots alive while everyone else got busy chasing reputation and revenue.

Just imagine, a clubhouse that feels more like your grandma's kitchen than a den of chaos. Pots clanging, meat on the stove, boots tracking in dirt, and laughter bouncing off the walls like children who never learned to use inside voices. Decisions aren't whispered behind doors by the three loudest men in the room. They're discussed over coffee, argued over like family, settled with handshakes and eye contact.

It's democracy but biker-style. Grease stains, bad jokes, and all.

These clubs don't need sponsorships or performative charity runs for clout.

They create meaning out of moments:

• the Sunday morning hangout after a long night
• the handshake that actually means "I've got you"
• the silent ride home after burying someone you loved

- the meals cooked because someone's fridge was empty
- the jokes told to keep someone from falling apart

That's the real MC world. The one no movie ever gets right.

Where Have I Taken on Shame That Doesn't Belong to Me?

Let's talk about shame. The kind that gets sewn onto you like a patch you never asked for.

Women in this world get judged harder than chrome on a hot day. Too loud. Too bold. Too sexual. Too opinionated. Too independent. Too emotional. Too quiet. Too something.

If you breathe too aggressively, somebody somewhere has something to say about it.

That's how misplaced shame creeps in. Sneaky as hell, like someone slipping a patch on your vest while you're not looking.

But here's the truth.
Most of that shame ain't yours. It belongs to the people who couldn't handle your fire.

It came from:
- men threatened by your voice
- outsiders judging what they don't understand
- other women repeating rules that were never written for us
- society deciding biker women are either saints or sluts. Nothing in between

I carried that weight for years.

Then I realized something. You can sell leather, but you can't buy legacy.

And the patch still belongs to the ones who bled for it. I'm done wearing shame stitched by other people's insecurities.

And if you're a woman reading this, you should be too.

The Candlelight Promise

Every candlelight ride is both a goodbye and a promise.

The goodbye is for the one we lost. The brother, the sister, the friend whose bike will never rumble again.

The promise is this.
You'll never ride alone.
Not in grief, not in life, not in the miles ahead.
That's the part outsiders don't get.

We are not villains.
We are not criminals.
We are not the stereotypes the news tries to paste on our backs.

But the world never stopped trying to make us the bad guys.
The women, especially.

So this part of Chapter 10? This is where we strip the chrome from the chaos and tell the truth. The real truth, about loyalty, legacy, and the way clubs can either save you or sell you out. And the difference between the two?

Heart.
Honor.
And who's sitting at the table when the votes are cast.

Chapter 10 Legacy Reflection Questions

1. Have you ever been part of a group or mission that lost its soul chasing money or power? What did it teach you about integrity, loyalty, or ego?

2. How do you personally balance the hustle of making money with staying true to your mission or code? Are there boundaries you've drawn, or need to?

3. What "brand" do you think you carry into the world? How does your outer image match (or clash with) your inner values?

4. Where do you draw the line between community and commerce?

5. Have you ever seen a group or friendship change when money gets involved? What did you learn?

PART III
CHROME, CHAOS & RECKONINGS

"Not all scars are visible.
Some ride under the skin,
rattling like loose bolts until you face them."

CHAPTER 11: CHROME & SHADOWS

"You don't just learn on the ride, you become on the ride."

Betrayal doesn't come with fists. It comes with silence. With a brother looking away when you need him most. With a sister who smiles at you one night, then whispers against you the next.

I've seen it burn down whole clubs. Not in the way Hollywood sells it gunfire, car bombs, shootouts in the desert but in the quiet moments. In the little cracks no one notices until the whole wall collapses.

*"The loudest wars don't happen between clubs.
They happen inside them."*

Trust is the currency of this world.
Code is the backbone.

And loyalty? That's the bloodline we swear on.

We talked about it back in Chapter 8. How this life is built on the idea that if you go down, somebody's gonna pick you up, patched or not. But here's the part nobody warns you about.

What happens when the trust breaks? What happens when the people who swore to protect you are the first to turn their backs?

I'll never forget one of those nights.

The clubhouse was packed, smoke hanging so thick you'd swear the walls were sweating. Conversations died mid-sentence. Boots scraped the floor as everyone shifted, waiting. When the vote was called, the energy in that room changed like someone turned the oxygen off.

A sister, someone I thought was rock-solid, stood in the center. She'd bled beside us. Laughed with us. Rode in storms with us. And now she was on trial for breaking the code.

No shouting.
No whiskey bottles flying.
Just the Sergeant-at-Arms stepping behind her and unfastening her patch.

The sound of those stitches ripping?

Slow. Final.

Like a heartbeat taking its last breath.

I will never forget the look in her eyes. Rage, shame, disbelief, all fighting for space. One minute you're wearing a legacy. The next you're standing in front of your family stripped bare. She walked out without a word, shoulders sagging under a weight only she understood.

That's betrayal in this world.
Not loud.
Not dramatic.
A quiet execution and it cuts deeper than any blade.

I've been in two women's clubs. Both built differently. Both taught me the same lesson:

The patch isn't the dangerous part.
People are.

And I've felt that silence in my own bones. The kind that comes when a sister you'd have died for looks at you like you're a stranger. When people you carried through hell let you burn alone. That pain doesn't heal. It just buries itself deeper and becomes part of your story, whether you want it or not.

Internal Conflict is the Real Club Killer

Forget the feds. Forget the headlines.

The truth is, most clubs don't fall because of law enforcement. People think clubs implode from the outside. Feds, rivals, raids. The truth? More often it's from within. Whispers, lies, broken trust and sometimes even worse.

I've watched strong chapters crumble not because of enemies, but because of egos. I've watched loyalty traded for power. I've watched good people leave broken because a bond they thought was unbreakable was tossed aside in a single vote. I have seen some become some broken they become a threat to themselves.

What if you're cruising with your friends on a road trip under a setting sun, laughing about old scars and sharing stories from the past. Sounds perfect, right?

Most clubs collapse from the inside.
I've watched chapters fall apart not because of enemies but because of egos.
Conflicts that started as whispers spread like gasoline on dry grass.

A president gets drunk on power.
A treasurer skims off the top.
A brother rats to save his own skin.
A patch is pulled in public, and the fallout splits the family in half.

The damage isn't just physical.
It's emotional. Spiritual. Generational.
That's what outsiders don't understand

betrayal doesn't just break a person.
 It haunts an entire club.

I've seen men walk away broken, not because of the streets, but because the club hurt them worse than any enemy could.

The silent betrayals. The manipulations.

In any brotherhood, there's an unspoken code that holds you together. You ride together, bleed together, and, most importantly, trust each other to have your back when times get tough. But what happens when that bond starts to weaken? When brotherly love shifts into bitter rivalry?

The decisions made in secret and sold as "brotherhood."

We don't talk enough about the grief in this lifestyle.
Yes there is grief.

And it absolutely deserves to be named. It's like watching a family cookout devolve into a chaotic food fight! Decisions made in secrecy, disguised as acts of brotherhood, can quickly spiral into betrayal.

The grief in this lifestyle is real, a heavy burden that many try to ignore. It lingers in the shadows, unspoken but ever-present.

When I think about broken bonds that still shape my self-worth, a few things come to mind. First off, let's talk about loyalty, the kind that feels like a second skin among your crew. When those bonds break, it can hit hard. It's not just about losing friends; it's about questioning your own value. Did I give too much? Did I trust the wrong people? Those thoughts sneak in and try to rewrite my worth. But here's the truth: real strength isn't found in never being hurt; it's in getting back on that bike after a wipe-out.

Then there are family ties, those sticky webs of love and obligation. Sometimes, family can be the toughest crowd, the ones who might never understand the biker code or what it means to be an 'Ol'Lady.' The judgments sting, and when you feel cast aside, it makes you wonder if you're enough. But this is where wisdom kicks in. I've chosen my tribe. They see me for who I am, a fierce spirit with a heart full of passion.

Every woman who rides knows this struggle. We've faced our share of "rules" and "codes," often made by those who don't truly understand what it means to be part of this biker family. You get labeled, banned, or pushed aside based on choices you didn't even make. But here's where things change, we learn to rewrite our own rules.

Broken friendships sting like a fresh tattoo gone wrong. They remind us of times when we felt invisible, lost among the noise of loud engines and bigger egos. Those moments can twist your self-worth into knots, making you question if you're worthy of respect or love. Yet, within that chaos lies an incredible opportunity for growth. Instead of allowing these wounds to define us, we flip the script.

Think about it, each scar tells a story of survival, showing how far we've come. Turn off the TV. If you want the truth, it's right here scarred, messy, and real.

My Own Crossroads

I know because I've felt it myself.

The night betrayal touched me, it wasn't a gun to the head, it was a look in the eyes of someone I trusted, suddenly cold, like I'd turned into a stranger. That silence told me everything.

I walked out of that clubhouse knowing the cut of betrayal is slow, deep, and permanent.

But here's what I also learned. Survival is in knowing when to ride away. Because sometimes loyalty to yourself is the only thing that saves you.

The Long Ride Lessons

- Loyalty will get tested.
- Betrayal will come from places you never expect.
- Sometimes the bravest thing you can do is stand your ground.
- Other times, it's walking away before the poison kills you too.

Either way, every betrayal leaves a mark. A scar you carry on the long ride. And every scar has a story.

Betrayal taught me this. Patches can be pulled, families can be fractured but the one bond you can't afford to break is with yourself.

Behind every stereotype are the scars. And those scars tell war stories louder than any rumor ever could. They are stories of resilience and strength, of finding light in the darkest moments. Each scar becomes a testament to the battles fought and the lessons learned. It's a reminder that while others may falter in their loyalty, staying true to oneself is the greatest triumph of all.

Chapter 11 Legacy Reflection Questions

1. Have you ever had to choose between loyalty to others and loyalty to yourself?

2. What's the deepest betrayal you've faced from someone you once trusted like family? Did it harden you, or teach you to set different boundaries?

3. Have you ever walked away from something that used to feel like "home"? Why did you leave, and how did you rebuild?

4. What does healing look like for you when your tribe fractures or the ride gets rough? Do you go quiet? Loud? Reflective? Revengeful? Real talk.

CHAPTER 12: WAR STORIES & WOUNDS

"Beauty and breakdown, we carry both."

If you think motorcycle clubs are all about brotherhood, bonfires, and maybe the occasional loud engine rev; well, it's way messier under that leather vest. Once you patch in, you're not just a rider; you're playing a high-stakes game of three-dimensional chess... except half the pieces want to stab you in the back.

"Every patch has a story. Every wound has a price."

People like to glamorize biker life. The leather, the brotherhood, the chrome catching sunlight on open roads. But the real battlefield isn't the pavement.

It's the politics. The power plays. The unspoken rules that hit harder than any bar fight.

I've seen grown men lose their minds over votes. I've watched loyalty twist into currency, respect turn into leverage. Everyone thinks the danger comes from the road, but the real explosions happen behind closed clubhouse doors. One wrong word can detonate a whole chapter. One ego can set a room on fire.
And while the men are busy chest-thumping and power climbing, the women, the Ol' Ladies, the supporters, the sisters, we're the ones who feel the tremors first. Women can sense when a room shifts. We know when something is off before the men even smell smoke. We feel the politics in our bones.

Because when walls shake?
We're the ones still standing when the dust settles.

But the politics don't stay inside the club.
They follow us into the world.

THE DAY MY CLOTHES BECAME A CRIME

Here's something that still stings, even after all the storms I've survived:

You walk into a bar, a restaurant, a VFW just trying to grab dinner, celebrate a birthday, support a fundraiser and suddenly someone half your size with none of your history steps up and chirps,

"Sorry, no colors allowed in here."

And what they mean is:
"We don't know you, but we're scared of the patch on your back."

Most of these people couldn't tell a club from a cartoon. They lump everyone with a hoodie, a vest, or a symbol into the same bucket, dangerous, trouble, not welcome.

Meanwhile, they don't know I've spent 23 years serving public safety, helping the very people who call me a risk. They don't know the fundraising rides I've led, the families I've helped bury loved ones, the cancer patients we've raised thousands for. They don't know the mothers I've stood beside, the veterans we've fed, or the kids we buy Christmas gifts for every damn year.

All they see is a piece of fabric.
A hoodie.
A word.
A color.

And just like that, I'm labeled a problem.

Let me clarify; I'm not angry; I'm disappointed. Disappointed that in 2025, people still judge others by their "cover" rather than the stories beneath.
My attire isn't a threat; it's a testimony. It represents loyalty woven into fabric.
If someone took the time to ask, I would explain;

"My colors represent charity, service, family, and the people I've stood beside through hell. If you're judging me by a hoodie, you're missing the whole damn point."
This is why I speak on it.   Not to rant but to educate.

To make people pause and think before they reduce a whole life to a stereotype.

The Night the Road Turned Black

There was a night that rewired something in me. Broke something open I didn't even know I had fortified.

Not because of the crash itself, but because of all the shadows that came after it. We were leaving a charity event, the kind where the kids hug you like you're made of magic and the parents thank you like you pulled them from the flames. We'd delivered toys, paid for a funeral meal, hugged strangers who felt more like family. The kind of night that reminds you why this lifestyle is worth bleeding for.

But the road... the road doesn't care about your good deeds.

Fog rolled in like a warning, thick and wet, clinging to the asphalt. You could taste the cold metal in the air. I remember thinking it felt like riding through a lung. Heavy, tight, alive in all the wrong ways. But we kept going, because that's what you do when you've got miles to eat.

Then the truck came.

Out of nowhere.
No lights.
No warning.
Just a wall of steel drifting into our lane like death on autopilot.

I saw the brother two bikes ahead of me hit the guardrail.
Not crash.
Hit.

The sound was... not a sound humans should hear.
Metal on bone.
Bone on steel.
Steel on pavement.

He flew.
I mean flew. His bike cartwheeling behind him, sparks slicing through the fog like fireworks.

The truck didn't stop. Didn't slow down. Didn't even acknowledge he existed.

While the world will paint bikers as the danger, that night proved something ugly.

Sometimes the real threat is a man too drunk to see the lives he's mowing down.

We pulled off hard, tires sliding. My back wheel fishtailed so violently I felt my ribs slam the tank. But adrenaline carries you through what common sense would never allow.

We found him half off the road, half in a ditch, his leg bent like wet paper, his breathing ragged. His cut was torn. Half off his body, the back panel ripped like someone had tried to erases his identity. There was so much blood I couldn't tell where it ended and the earth began.

I dropped to my knees beside him, gravel slicing through my jeans, cold mud swallowing my boots. His eyes were open but vacant. Like he was somewhere between here and whatever waits in the dark on the other side.

I held his head.

He didn't know it was me at first.

He kept whispering, "Don't take my patch. Don't take my patch."

That wreck didn't scare him.
The idea of dying without his identity did.

We used belts, bandanas, whatever we had. One of the guys ripped his T-shirt off with his teeth because his hands were shaking too hard to grip the fabric. We were covered in blood and oil and fog and fear. You don't forget that mix. It sinks into your skin.

The silence before the sirens was the longest ten minutes of my life.
When they finally arrived, the paramedics hovered, reluctant, like we were danger instead of the only reason he was still breathing.

Then came the cops.
And their questions.
And their assumptions.
And the way they looked at the patch like it was a criminal record.

"Are these your colors?"
"What's he affiliated with?"
"Any drugs or weapons on the bikes?"

Not one:
"Is your friend dying?"
Later at the ER, they refused to let his vest stay on the bed. The nurse said, "No gang attire," like we'd walked in spraying bullets instead of holding a man's artery shut for ten miles.

I stood there wearing jeans soaked in his blood while they treated us like the threat.

That's the wound.
Not the visible ones.
Not the fractures or scars.

But the deep, quiet ache of knowing,
We saved a life that night.
And the world still treated us like the villains.

When I went home hours later, I sat on my garage floor with my helmet still on, unable to peel myself out of the moment.

There's a darkness that comes with this life.
Not the Hollywood bullshit.
Not gun deals or shootouts.

But this, The darkness of loving people the world hates. The darkness of knowing the road can take anyone at any time.

The darkness of watching a brother beg not to lose his identity while bleeding out.

It changed me.
It made me sharper.
Colder in some ways.
Softer in others.

It taught me that loyalty is a blessing and a curse and that the world will judge your leather long before it ever sees your humanity.

That night tattooed a truth into my bones. We are more than the stories they tell about us.

And the road doesn't take the ones who deserve it.
It takes the ones who ride.

The Shift: From Politics to Power

Out there in the world, as inside the club, people assume a lot about women like me.

They expect softness without strength.
Silence without wisdom.
Support without self-respect.

But here's the truth I had to grow into,
Desire starts with how you see yourself.
If you don't honor your own worth, everyone else will treat you like a discount version of who you could be.
I learned that the hard way.

Not through fairy tales through fire, betrayal, bar fights, funerals, and empty rooms that taught me who would really show up.

When you love yourself, you stop accepting:
- half-assed loyalty
- shady energy
- men who only show up in the dark
- people who want your presence but not your peace

You learn to stand tall in your own damn patch, even when you're not wearing one.

When Power Devours

Power is funny.
It doesn't just corrupt, it consumes.

In club life, in work life, in relationships, anywhere men gather in a hierarchy, there's always someone ready to climb over someone else to feel taller.

I've seen it:
Men who want control but not responsibility.
Men who want followers but not accountability.
Men who want the title but none of the sacrifice.

And women?
We get caught in the crossfire unless we choose a different path.

So I chose mine;
I stopped asking for space and started claiming it.
Respect isn't something you wait for, it's something you live loud enough to make undeniable.

The Truth About Wounds

The deepest wounds in this life aren't the bloody ones.

They're the ones you carry quietly;
- The betrayal that blindsides you.
- The room that judges you without knowing you.
- The friend who vanishes when your illness gets loud.
- The man who calls you "strong" but never stays long enough to see why.

Every woman in biker culture carries her own war stories.
And every one of them deserves to be told without shame.
These aren't just stories.
They are survival maps.
They are proof.
And they are the reason I write so no woman feels like she's the only one bleeding behind the scenes.

Chapter 12 Legacy Reflection Questions

1. Where have you been judged by the outside instead of the truth in your heart?

2. What wound shaped you the most and what strength did it give you?

3. Who taught you the cost of loyalty, and what did it take to finally understand your own worth?

4. What are you still carrying that deserves to be set down?

CHAPTER 13: STORM BORN – ILLNESS, IDENTITY, AND THE COST OF STRENGTH

"You can be the storm and still have soft bones."

Forget what you've heard, charity in the biker world isn't just men writing checks. Some of the fiercest acts of service I've seen came from the women who refused to let anyone fall through the cracks.

I didn't become a storm because I wanted to.
I became one because life wouldn't stop striking.

Illness came at me like lightning. Fast, bright, merciless.

Cancer. MS. Lupus. A trifecta of hell that didn't knock…
 just kicked the damn door in and made itself at home.

You don't get time to prepare.
You don't get a handbook.
You don't get a gentle introduction.

You get a diagnosis.
Then another.
Then another.

And suddenly the woman you were dies slowly while the woman you're becoming claws her way up from the wreckage.

Charity Isn't Just for the Men

People outside the biker world love to tell stories about what they think our life looks like. Like we're all tattoos, trouble, and turf. What they never talk about are the women holding communities together with bare hands and medical bottles.

One winter, a widow in our circle was drowning.
Rent overdue. Kids hungry. Heat cut off.

Brotherhood arguing over how to help while she was quietly falling apart.

The women didn't hesitate.
We didn't need a vote.
We didn't need permission.
We didn't need a committee.

By sunrise, flyers were out.
By noon, donations poured in.
By the weekend, the clubhouse was shoulder-to-shoulder with people feeding her kids, paying her bills, and reminding her she wasn't alone.

That's the part nobody sees. The women holding the damn sky up. We're the storm shelters. We're the ground crews. We rebuild the town while the men ride through the wreckage.

The Storm That Moved Into My Body

Illness isn't polite.
It doesn't knock.
It just barges in and rearranges your entire life like it pays the mortgage.

The real betrayal wasn't the pain. It was the way people disappeared. I had plenty of friends but not many who stayed to watch a movie or help with my wheelchair.

Not many who saw me collapse on the floor.

Not many who heard me say, "I don't think I can do this anymore." And stayed anyway.
That's the loneliness no doctor warns you about.

Illness showed me who I could trust.
Club life showed me who I absolutely couldn't.

Some days my joints felt like rusted bolts.

Some days my skin felt like it was trying to escape my bones.
Some days breathing felt like work.

People told me I "looked good now."
As if looking good meant I wasn't fighting for every minute of my life.

The Night My Body Became a Battlefield

One night after a club event, the weather turned on me like it had been waiting for its cue.
A storm rolled in fast. Black clouds, bone-rattling rain, the kind that makes the world feel too small.

I should've stayed at the event we were hosting.
I should've waited.

But illness teaches you this toxic lie.
If I don't keep up, I'll get left behind.

Halfway home, the pain hit.
Not a flare.
A full-body mutiny.

My hands locked on the throttle.

My legs trembled so hard I could feel the bike shifting under me. My vision narrowed until the road looked like a tunnel about to swallow me whole.

I pulled off right at the stop sign, rain soaking through my leather and my clothes until they felt like weights dragging me down.

I sat there on my bike, shaking, burning, sobbing, unable to lift myself.

And you want to know the part that cracked me open?
Not that I was in pain.
Not that I was alone.
Not even that I thought I was about to die in a puddle on the side of the road.

It was that I didn't want to call anyone.

Because I didn't know who would answer.
Because illness had already shown me the truth. Most people only show up when the weather is good.

But that night, someone did come.

My daughter. Barely on a bike before, she knew I need her.

She didn't ask for details.
She didn't make a speech.
She didn't judge.

She just held me up and said, "You're not dying tonight. Not on my watch."

Sometimes storms don't just break you.
They introduce you to moments that will rebuild you.

Identity in the Aftermath

Illness stripped away everyone who loved the easy version of me.
The fun version.
The strong version.

The woman who didn't need help.

What was left was raw.
Soft.
Scared.
Real.

I stopped chasing approval.
I stopped explaining myself.
I stopped apologizing for the fire people couldn't handle.

I rebuilt myself with boundaries, honesty, and the kind of faith you earn through suffering.

If I could talk to the woman I was before the diagnoses, I'd tell her this:
"You don't break easy. You bend. And everything that tries to drown you will one day bow to the woman you become."

Soft Bones, Hard Battles

Survivors, empaths, and women of faith, listen close.

Your softness is not weakness.
Your tears are not a failure.
Your boundaries are not selfish.

You can be gentle and still be a warrior.
You can be vulnerable and still be powerful.
You can be sick and still be unstoppable.

You don't heal by becoming someone new.
You heal by coming home to the warrior you always were.

Give yourself the grace you've poured into others. Let go of the ones who loved you only when it was easy. And remember you are allowed to take up space, even in your most fragile form.

That whisper is where I met my true self.

Not in the noise of a crowded bar. Not on a patch worn proudly by bikers. And definitely not just hanging off the back of a motorcycle.

Letter to the Woman I Was

Sometimes surviving looks like resting without guilt.

Before I step into the next part of my story, I need to speak to the woman I used to be.

The one I almost lost.
The one who fought the hardest battles alone.
This is for her.

Chapter 13 Legacy Reflection Questions

1. Who am I still trying to be strong for, and what would it look like to be strong for myself?

2. Who stood by you during your most painful moments, and who disappeared? What did that teach you about the relationships you want moving forward?

3. What would you say to the version of yourself who didn't know if she'd make it through?

4. How do you define strength today, and how has that definition changed since your diagnosis?

Pit Stop #4 — Handlebar Attitudes

You've just survived a chorus of engine revs, gruff nods, and unsolicited advice from a biker who's convinced that handlebars have a "no women allowed" sign painted on them. Time for a pit stop. Here's where you pull over, kick back with a metaphorical cup of coffee, and say something like, "Ah yes, the macho biker brigade, proof that some men think the only thing more intimidating than a roaring Harley is a confident woman owning the road.

These encounters are less about handlebars and more about handlebar attitudes, reminding us that the fight for female visibility isn't just in boardrooms or political rallies. Sometimes, it's revving loudly next to you at the stoplight, insisting that the cultural terrain is as bumpy as the backroads we ride."

Letter to the Woman I Was,

Letter to the Woman I Was.

Dear Me — the woman I was, the woman who almost didn't make it,
I see you.

Alone.

Hooked up to beeping machines in another cold hospital room.
Trying to make peace with pain while pretending you're not scared.

It's 3am, and the silence is screaming.

You're too exhausted to cry, too stubborn to ask for help.
You hate what your body has become.
You hate that this is what surviving looks like.

But hear me clearly:
You are not weak.
You are not broken.
You are not too much.
You are the storm.

Life handed you sharp edges. Diagnoses that steal your sense of safety, Friends who disappeared the moment your strength wasn't convenient, people who called you tough "just so they didn't have to show up."

And still... here you are.

Strength isn't always loud.

Sometimes it's crawling instead of roaring.
Sometimes it's resting without guilt.
Sometimes it's whispering......
"I matter even when I'm not okay."

There were nights the pain felt predatory.
Days MS and Lupus dragged you under.
Moments when your own skin betrayed you and your mind spiraled.

You kept asking, "Will I ever feel normal again?"

Baby girl...
you were never meant to be normal.
You were born for the edge of the storm.

People see your fire now, the laugh, the leather, the patch, the road beneath your boots,
but they don't know the cost.

They don't know the migraines that stole your mornings.

They don't know how many times you grieved the older, healthier version of yourself.

They don't know how you built boundaries like barbed wire, not because you wanted to push love away, but because you were done being hurt.

But I know.

And I am proud of you.

You stopped chasing people who made you feel too hard to love.

You started giving your energy to people who matched your heart and your faith.

You stopped trying to earn worth.

You finally started walking in it.

The woman in that hospital bed didn't die there.

She rose.

And when she did, she became me!

HelKat

CHAPTER 14: WOMEN WHO RIDE; FAITH IN THE REARVIEW

"God didn't forget me, He just gave me a backbone first."

By the time most people knew me as HelKat, I'd already been through wars no one could see. Cancer. Lupus. MS. Each one tried to steal pieces of me; my strength, my rhythm, even my identity.

Faith in the Rearview

"God didn't forget me... He just gave me grit first."

By the time most people knew me as HelKat, the loud one with the patched-up leather, the quick tongue, and the backbone welded from steel, I'd already survived wars nobody saw. Not club wars. The kind that happen in hospital beds, in quiet bathrooms where you brace yourself against the sink, in the spaces between breath and breakdown.

People love to talk about "strength, but they don't talk about the price.

Chapter Three showed the fight in the chemo chair. Those cold floors, those whispering nurses, those beeping machines that marked time like a countdown. But nobody tells you what comes after. Nobody prepares you for the part where survival becomes a second job.

Because the truth is this,

Survival doesn't end when treatment ends. Survival begins when everyone else thinks you're "better."

They see the color coming back to your cheeks.

They see the smile reappearing.

They see you out at dinner again, maybe riding again, maybe laughing again.

What they don't see are the things I had to make peace with in private:
- mornings where my legs refused to cooperate
- the way my hands shook pouring a cup of coffee
- nights when my bones screamed like they were lined with broken glass
- the shame of canceling plans because my body staged a protest
- the fear of waking up the next day and not recognizing myself in my own skin

Everyone applauds your strength...
...but no one sees the bill.

That's the betrayal of illness. **Your body is still fighting long after the world stops clapping.**

My Mother Taught Me What Strength Really Looks Like

If I learned grit from illness, I learned **grace** from my mother. She was always loud like me. She is Italian and always flashy and the type to slam doors or curse the sky. She will fight her own battles with a dignity that could break your heart.

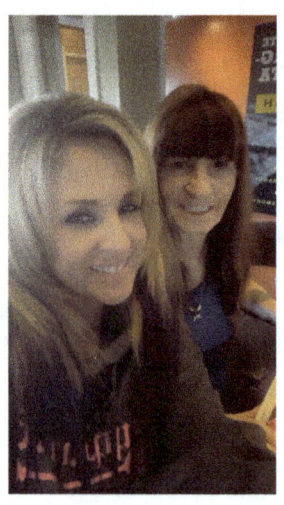

I remember one night she was weak, pale, and too tired to stand on her own.
I wrapped my arm around her to help her into bed, and she whispered,

"Don't rush me. Let me do as much as I can."

It wasn't pride.
                      It was purpose.

She wanted to feel alive in whatever pieces she had left.
That moment stayed with me.

Because later, when MS and lupus tried to take my independence, I heard her voice in the back of my mind saying, *"Let me do as much as I can."*

And I did.
Even when it hurt.
Even when I was scared.
Even when the world thought I should crumble.

She didn't just teach me how to survive illness, she taught me how to survive myself.

When she got sick, when cancer stole her strength, I watched a woman who weighed barely eighty-something pounds still fight like she had thunder in her blood.

I remember sitting on the floor beside her recliner one night.
She was too weak to speak much, too tired to pretend she wasn't hurting. The house was quiet. The kind of quiet that feels like it's listening.

She took my hand, squeezed with what little strength she had left, and said:

"Baby... don't you ever quit your life trying to survive someone else's pain."

I also inherited something from her that night no illness could ever take:

Her fire. Her fighter's heart. Her quiet, relentless faith.

My survival is her victory too.
That's the real war, not the pain but the identity crisis.

Your body changes.
Your limits change.
Your pace changes.
Your people change.

The Ride That Should've Broke Me (But Didn't)

There was a night late fall, sky thick with the kind of cold that slices through leather when I took my bike out during an MS flare because staying home felt like surrender. My legs were shaking before I even hit the main road. I could barely squeeze the clutch. My palms were slick with sweat, but not the good kind. The fear kind.

Halfway to the house, my hands went numb.

Not tingly but gone.

I pulled over on a dark back road, hands gripping the bars like they were the only thing keeping me tethered to the earth. My vision blurred. I felt my body slipping out from under me.

I swear to you, right there under a dead streetlight, I whispered it myself, *"Not tonight. You can take my legs, but you're not taking my ride."*

I sat there until the numbness retreated enough to move. I rode home slow, shaking, praying, promising God I'd stop being stubborn, a promise we both knew I'd break.

That night taught me something no doctor, pastor, or patch holder ever could, The storm wasn't killing me. It was forging me.

I grieved versions of me that will never return.

The woman with boundless energy, no scars, no fear of waking up broken.

But healing isn't becoming someone new.
Healing is coming home to the warrior you've always been.

Boundaries, Not Apologies

Illness taught me the word that saved my life:

No.

No to pushing myself past breaking.
No to being small to keep someone else comfortable.
No to letting anyone mistake my strength for silence.

My body may betray me,
but I refuse to betray myself ever again.

Boundaries rebuilt me.
Faith steadied me.
And the road reminded me who I am.

Because if I had to choose between being "easy to love" and being real?
I'll take real every time.

And you're left standing in the wreckage asking,
"Who am I now?"

I'll tell you who!
You're the woman who learned how to live inside a body that doesn't always cooperate.

You're the woman who knows her worth even when her legs go numb.

You're the woman who built boundaries the world never taught her how to hold.

You're the woman who gets back on the bike even when it feels like betrayal.

This chapter isn't just about illness.

It's about the moment you stop surviving for other people...
and start surviving for yourself.
And baby, that's where the magic begins.

Where Biker Life Meets Survival

Outsiders see chaos, noise, rebellion.

But here's the truth,
Biker life teaches survival the same way illness does.

Both demand that you:
- know your limits
- trust your tribe
- stand your ground
- live like time isn't guaranteed
- build strength in the dark
- find peace in the roar

The road and the chemo chair look nothing alike but both made me who I am.

Both broke me open.
Both showed me truth.
Both taught me to fight for breath.
Both taught me that life isn't meant to be quiet.

And both taught me this,
You get one ride.
Make it loud enough to hear over the storms.

Illness taught me how to survive myself.
But biker sisterhood?
That taught me how to survive the world.

And that's where the next chapter begins;
with the women who held me together
when everything else tried to pull me apart.

Chapter 14 Legacy Reflection Questions

1. What did survival look like after your hardest season, not during it?

2. Where in your life have you kept going when your body or spirit said stop?

3. What is one boundary you need to set to protect your energy and healing?

4. Who is a woman whose strength shaped your own and what did she teach you?

5. What freedom are you ready to reclaim, even if it must be done slowly, painfully, or loudly?

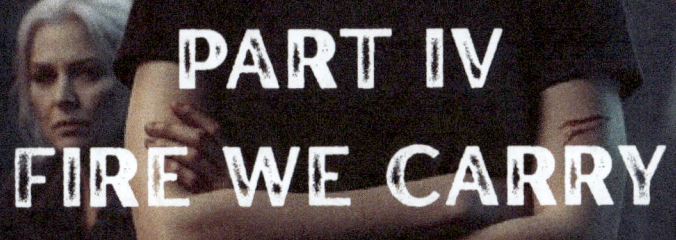

PART IV
FIRE WE CARRY

"We're not just keeping the fire alive.
We are the fire —
and it burns loud enough to outlive us all."

CHAPTER 15: MOTHERS, MATRIARCHS & THE FIRE WE CARRY

"I was never strong, I was surviving. There's a difference."

The matriarchs of the biker world don't always wear patches, but they sure as hell carry the weight. These women are the unsung anchors: biker moms, biker wives, biker sisters, the keepers of order, the voice of reason, the ride-or-dies who make sure the family keeps rolling. Whether raising kids in a clubhouse, running fundraising events, or nursing wounded egos and busted knuckles, these women are fierce, funny, and often forgotten. It's time they got their spotlight.

The matriarchs of the biker world don't always wear patches.

Most of the time, they don't wear anything that marks them at all. But you can spot them a mile away by the way people move toward them in chao and the way they never ask for anything in return.

These women are the quiet anchors. Biker moms, wives, sisters, the fixers, the planners, the ones who remember every birthday and every bail hearing.

They hold the line while everyone else rides the storm. And somewhere along the way, without ceremony or applause, I became one of them.

I didn't choose that role.

Life shoved it into my hands like hot iron.

Motherhood taught me how to endure.
The clubhouse taught me how to lead.
Survival taught me how to carry fire without burning everything down.

But the night I knew I was the matriarch?
It wasn't dramatic.
It wasn't glamorous.

It was 2AM, barefoot, hair wild, looking through the peephole at a girl crying on my porch.

The Night They Came to My Door

I'll never forget that knock.
Not the gentle kind.

Not the "you up?" kind.

No! This was a panic-pound, the kind that rattles the doorframe and your soul.

I opened it and there she was. A prospect's girlfriend, mascara streaked, hoodie half-off, shaking so hard I thought she'd fall forward into my arms.

"HelKat... I didn't know where else to go."

Translation - I created chaos, and now I need someone else to clean it up.

She'd already called the cops.
Already filed the report.
Already said she wanted a PFA.
But now?
Now she wanted me to play Uber for her to go confront him.

Girl.
No. Absolutely not.

I stood there in my doorway, looking at this tornado in sweatpants, thinking, why do these women always show up when the paperwork is already filed?

She begged.
She pleaded.
She wanted me to "just drive her over there so he'd understand."

Understand WHAT?
She'd already lit the fuse and then wanted me to hold the bomb.

I wasn't sacrificing safety, sanity, or sleep because someone else didn't know how to leave cleanly.

So I looked her dead in the eyes and said,
"Baby, I will help you calm down.

I will help you plan your next step.

But I'm not driving you into a fight you already started.

She cried harder.
But she knew I meant it.

That night taught me the difference between helping and enabling.

Between protection and puppetry.
Between being a mother and being a martyr.

And for the first time, I realized,

People come to the matriarch not because she's weak, but because she's the only one who won't lie to them.

I didn't drive her anywhere.
I made her tea, sat her at my table, and told her truths she didn't want to hear.

Truths no one ever told me when I needed them.
When the sun came up, she walked away calmer and I walked back into my room, exhausted but steady.

Because sometimes the fire you carry isn't anger, it's clarity.

The Mother I Became Because I Had To

Being a mother in this world isn't soft.
It's survival with mascara and a mouth that knows how to pray and cuss at the same time.

But here's the moment that broke me open. I was hiding in the bathroom. Door locked, hand over my mouth because I didn't want my daughters to see me cry again.

My joints were screaming.
My nerves were on fire.

I had just spent fifteen minutes cooking dinner with one hand on the counter because the pain hit so hard I couldn't stand up straight.

But I didn't want them to think
"Mom is sick again."

So I kept stirring the damn pot like nothing was wrong.
Then I heard it.
Soft.
Small.
From the hallway.

"Mom… it's okay. We know you're trying."
That was the moment I realized, I wasn't just their mother.

I was their blueprint. Their first example of a woman who bends but doesn't break. Who fights but still loves. Who hurts but still gets dinner on the table.

I never wanted my daughters to grow up knowing pain like mine. But I damn sure wanted them to grow up knowing strength like mine.

Strength that isn't hardness.
Strength that isn't silence.
Strength that isn't martyrdom.

The kind of strength that whispers,

"You're allowed to rest. You're allowed to feel. You're allowed to take up space."

The Matriarchs Before Us

Matriarchs aren't the loudest voices.

They're the ones who can hear a lie in a whisper. They're the ones people call at midnight when the world has fallen apart. They're the ones who hold traditions and trauma in the same hands and somehow make it look easy.

Biscuit taught me to laugh through chaos.
Santa taught me to give without expecting anything back.
Redman taught me that legacy matters more than loudness.

And the women
oh, the women
they taught me everything else.

How to heal.
How to love.
How to run a home and a fundraiser simultaneously.
How to survive in a world built for men but held together by women.

What I Want My Daughters to Know

I don't want them to be perfect.
I want them to be powerful.

I don't want them to be fearless.
I want them to ride anyway.
I don't want them to avoid storms.
I want them to become them.

Because that's the legacy we pass down behind the patch!
A road of resilience.
A map of survival.
And a fire that never goes out.

Some women inherit china sets and family recipes. My daughters will inherit a legacy built from grit, chrome, and the kind of love that shows up before sunrise with coffee and a plan.

They'll know what it means to stand their ground, to help without losing themselves, and to let their fire burn without apology.

Because the truth is simple, mothers carry fire, but matriarchs learn how to use it.

And baby; behind the patch, that makes all the difference.

Even when you've carried everyone else, even when you've cooked the meals, dried the tears, cleaned the blood, and held the line, you still have to face yourself in the end.
Motherhood teaches you how to show up for others.

Matriarchhood teaches you how to lead them. But healing? Healing teaches you how to come home to the version of you that was buried under all the survival.

And that's where the next chapter begins. The unraveling.

The quiet reckoning. The moment when the ride slows down long enough for you to hear your own heartbeat again.

Because after all the chaos, all the loyalty tests, all the funerals and fundraisers and kitchen-table war rooms, there comes a night when the house is finally quiet, the kids are asleep, and the storm you've been outrunning turns around and sits at your table.

And you have to decide if you're ready to stop surviving and start living.

That's Chapter 16.

The chapter where the road turns inward.

Where freedom stops being something you chase and starts being something you claim.

Chapter 15 Legacy Reflection Questions

1. Who are the women in your life who've held it all together behind the scenes? How do they lead without needing credit?

2. Have you ever downplayed your own power because you weren't "patched in"? What would it look like to own it instead?

3. What lessons do you want your children, or the next generation, to carry from you?

4. When was the last time you felt truly powerful in your own skin, despite the pain?

CHAPTER 16: BROTHERHOOD & BETRAYAL

"The cut on your back means nothing if the knife in mine came from you."

Since the dawn of black-and-white film reels, motorcycle clubs have been Hollywood's favorite boogeymen, like vampires, but with leather jackets and louder engines. More like the full-on monsters under the bed.

Hollywood has been chasing biker stories since the dawn of shaky black-and-white film reels. According to the screenwriters, we're either leather-clad vampires, highway terrorists, or the devil's sidekicks on two wheels. The media makes us look like monsters under the bed, just swap the fangs for cuts and chrome.

But here's the part the headlines never show, most motorcycle clubs aren't crime scenes on wheels.

They're families.
Messy, loud, loyal, dysfunctional as hell, yes! But families.

And when the world slaps a label on your back before you even walk through the door, that reputation becomes a second skin. Something you didn't choose, but have to drag around anyway. It sticks to you harder than road tar, and it damages real people in real ways. Jobs lost. Doors closed. Kids judged by last names and patches they didn't even earn.

People fear what they don't understand.

And what they don't understand, they stereotype.
And what they stereotype, they try to erase.

That kind of weight?
Even the strongest biker woman feels it in her bones.

But then there were the moments that were rare, unexpected, holy in their own crooked way. When I surrendered. Not to fear, not to judgment, but to something bigger. Something I can't fully define. God, the wind, the ancestors, the universe... take your pick. Whatever it was, it met me right where I was breaking.

Like that one ride.

Just me, my bike, and an endless strip of road that didn't give a damn about my club's reputation or my diagnoses. The sky cracked open wide enough for me to breathe again. The wind didn't just hit my face, it whispered,
"Let that shit go, girl."

For the first time in a long time, I loosened my grip.

Not on the handlebars, hell no, I can ride a straight line blindfolded but on the heaviness I'd been carrying. The betrayal from people who swore they'd die for me.

The disappointment of being judged by headlines instead of heart.

The fear of being erased by stories I didn't write.

The anger at being misunderstood by a world that only sees caricatures.

Letting go didn't make me weak. It made me dangerous in a different way.

Focused.
Soft in the right places. where it mattered.
Untouchable in others and everywhere else.

That's the truth about sisterhood and betrayal in this life. It's not always the bullets, the bar fights, or the patches that break you.

It's the story the world tells about you and the one you finally decide to tell for yourself.
And this chapter?
This is where I tell mine.

The Media Meat Grinder

Those Hollywood stories? They're as one-sided as a three-legged race.

TV shows, clickbait headlines, documentaries made by people who've never ridden a mile. They build myths that stick harder than grease on a chain.
And the damage?
Real.
Ugly.
Deep.

It's the kind of weight that makes even the toughest biker woman feel like she's dragging a damn boulder uphill while wearing six layers of leather. (And trust me, leather isn't lightweight. Especially in July.)

But every now and then, something bigger steps in. Something that reminds you you're more than the world's commentary.

But there were these rare, magical moments where I surrendered, not in defeat, but to something bigger. Like that one ride: just me and my bike beneath an endless sky. The wind wasn't just whipping through my hair, it was freedom whispering in my ear, saying, "Girl, lighten up."

Call it spirits, call it the universe, or that weird thing your grandma calls faith, there are forces out there that can actually help you unload. I'm not usually one for surrendering (my rebellious heart prefers to brawl), but after feeling lost, betrayed, and scared of being erased from the stories I wanted to live, I finally listened to that quieter voice inside me. That voice said, "Hey, maybe stop trying to keep every rule tattooed in your mind and just trust something bigger."

Picture this: It's late at night, the road unrolling endlessly like a breast cancer ribbon under my tires. Inside my head? Chaos. Curveballs flying like a bad poker hand (I don't know how to play poker) confessions of betrayal, the weight of loyalty, the legacy I was trying to uphold, and the gnawing question, "Am I even measuring up to the legends who came before me?". Suddenly, I'm not the tough biker woman everyone expects, I'm just a human, holding too much for any one pair of boots to carry (or should I say bra to hold, LOL)

That night, I parked my bike and looked up at the stars scattered like patches on our vests, each one telling a story thicker than a bar fight at midnight. And in that quiet moment, I realized something crucial, it's okay to admit when you need help. My legs are weak from the MS, my face burning from lupus and my heart pounding from sheer hell. Toughness doesn't mean never falling; sometimes, it means knowing when to lean on faith, whether you call it that or fate, or good old cosmic humor.

I've had my share of low points. I'm talking about life pitching curveballs so nasty they'd make even the toughest biker flinch, betrayals, doubts about loyalty, the ticking clock of being forgotten. I was so deep in survival mode, clinging to every code and rule like they were lifelines, I forgot to listen to that little, rebellious voice inside saying, "Hey, maybe trust something else for a change." Sounds a bit like hippie talk, I know, but when I finally leaned into that faith, whatever form it took, it was like suddenly I found a map through the chaos.

The media meat grinder might still try to chew us up and spit us out as villains, but here's the truth they'll never tell. MCs are warriors of loyalty, resilience, and sometimes downright stubborn faith. And for all the stereotypes flung our way, that's a legacy worth riding for.

Brotherhood is the word that gets thrown around the most in this life, painted on banners, shouted across rallies, etched into skin with ink and scar tissue. But brotherhood isn't the patches, or the toasts, or the ride photos on the wall. It's what you do when the storm hits. And betrayal? It shows up when the storm is loudest.

I've watched it play out in silence before it ever exploded. A brother avoiding your eyes. A phone call that goes unanswered one too many times. A pause too long before they say, "You know I've got your back."

And then one day, you realize they don't.

The Knife Behind the Patch

The night it happened to me, the clubhouse looked normal, smoke thick, laughter spilling out of every corner. But under it all, there was a wrongness. A sister I trusted, one I'd carried through her own hell, looked straight through me like I wasn't even there. Betrayal isn't always a scream. Sometimes it's a knife slipped between ribs with a smile still on the face.

That's the part the world doesn't see. They see the brawls, the raids, the mugshots. What they don't see is the quiet devastation when a bond breaks inside the circle. Fists heal. Broken bones mend. But trust? Once it's cracked, it never fits back the same.

When Brotherhood Shatters

I've seen men sworn in blood walk out when the heat got real. I've seen women left to clean up the wreckage after loyalty turned out to be just lip service. The cut you wear might mean family, but the knife still fits too easily in the hands of someone you once called "brother."

And when it happens, it guts you. It makes you question not just them, but yourself. How did I not see it? How did I not hear the silence growing?

The truth is, betrayal doesn't happen because you're weak. It happens because you chose to believe.

Brotherhood is holy, but betrayal is hell. And I've been through both.

So don't tell me loyalty is ink on skin. Don't tell me family is a patch. I've bled for both, and I know the truth;
The only bonds worth keeping are the ones that don't break when the fire starts.

When betrayal and grief stacked high, I turned to the only confessional that never let me down, the open road itself.

Chapter 16 Legacy Reflection Questions

1. What's the most damaging stereotype you've heard about bikers, and why do you think it persists?

2. How do you respond when someone gets your story wrong? Do you correct it, walk away, or rewrite it louder?

3. When someone gets your story hilariously wrong, do you straighten them out, walk away coolly, or crank your version up to eleven?

Pit Stop #5: The Tank Top Tango

Show up to a biker meet in a tank top and you'll get all kinds of "Are you serious?" glances. But here's the thing: while some see exposed arms as a challenge to the tough biker aesthetic, I see them as a spotlight on the unspoken battle for visibility. Because nothing says, "I belong here" like defying the unwritten dress code designed by the 'old guard.' Plus, sunburn beats invisibility any day.

Feminist Flash: Your wardrobe is your first skirmish in claiming space, even if it's just the right to rock a tank top without sideways stares.

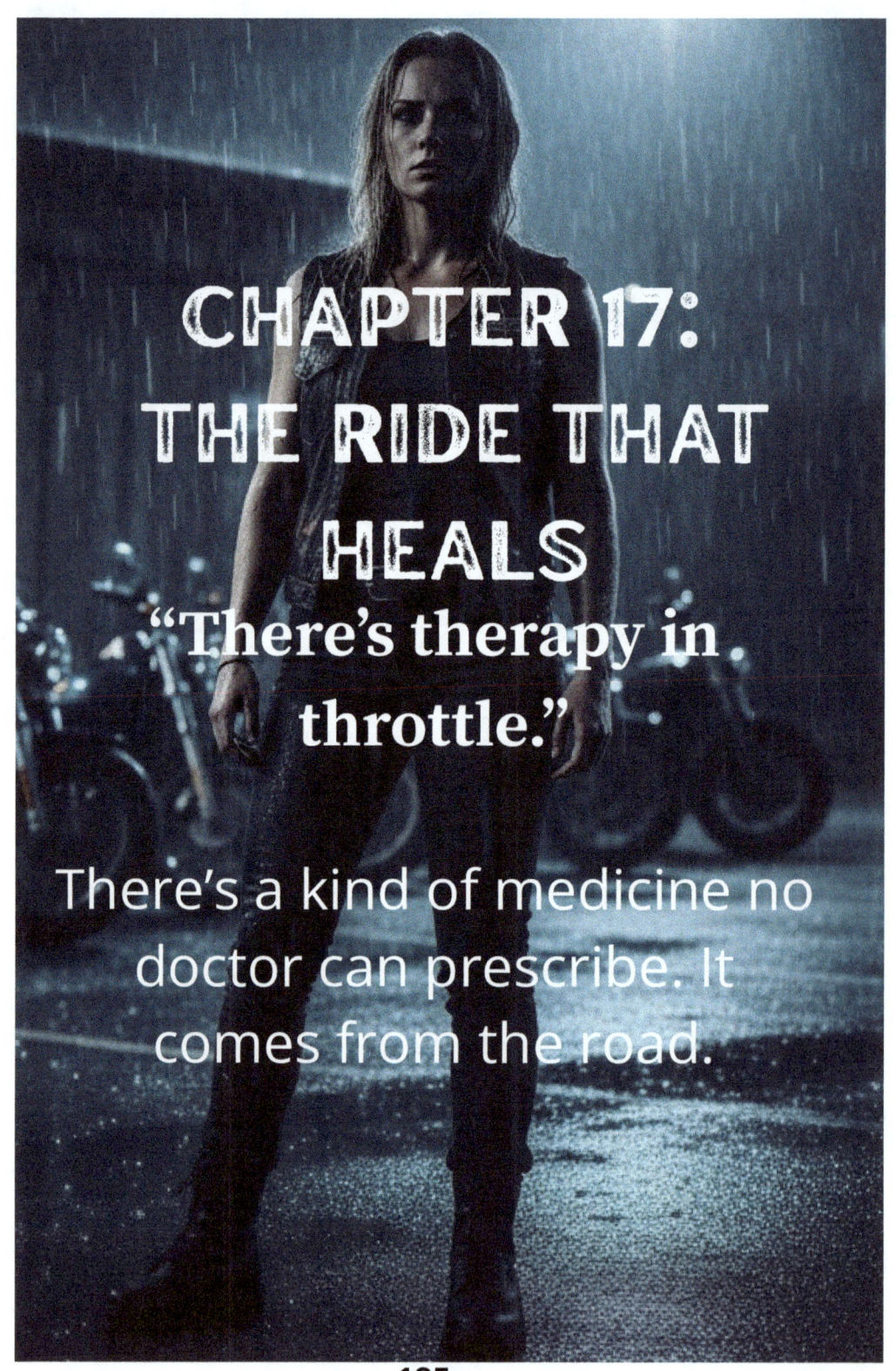

CHAPTER 17: THE RIDE THAT HEALS

"There's therapy in throttle."

There's a kind of medicine no doctor can prescribe. It comes from the road.

I've ridden with tubes still taped to my arm, hair barely grown back from chemo, body aching in ways most people will never know. And yet, when I ride my bike and fire the engine, something shifts. Pain doesn't disappear but it falls back, like a shadow that can't keep up with the light.

The roar of the pipes drowns out the noise in my head. The vibration rattles loose the grief that gets stuck in my chest. Out there, I don't have to explain myself. I don't have to be the sick woman, the single mom, the ol' lady, the survivor. I just get to be me.

I've cried behind my shades, helmet tilted back so the tears could ride the wind instead of my cheeks. I've screamed into the night sky with only the stars as my witness. I've whispered the names of people I've lost, letting the wind carry them where I couldn't.

The road doesn't judge. It listens.

And every time I come back from a ride, I'm lighter. Not healed, maybe, but unburdened.

For some, a ride is rebellion. For me, it's resurrection. Every mile feels like prayer. Every curve is a sermon. Every sunrise caught from the saddle is proof that life is still worth showing up for.

Grief, trauma and illness ride with me, but they don't drive anymore. The throttle is mine. The freedom is mine. The road reminds me I'm alive, and that's holy enough.

For many of us, wind therapy isn't a trend, it's survival. We talk about grief, loss, trauma, and how two wheels and an open road have helped thousands of rider's process pain in ways therapy never touched. We explore memorial rides, suicide prevention efforts, and how riding becomes a spiritual act of release. Memorial rides, poker runs, are the kind of soul-cleansing that only a long, open highway can deliver all prove that riding isn't just a hobby, it's therapy dressed in leather and gasoline fumes.

Which Scars Am I Ready to Wear with Pride Instead of Pain

Alright, let's break it down. Scars aren't just marks on our skin; they're stories carved into us, proof that we've faced battles and come out stronger. Think about the moments in your life that shaped you.

We are talking about pain and healing that left scars. No, not the ones that make your skin look like a well-mapped treasure chart (though those are cool too), but the ones embedded deep in your story. Scars aren't just ugly souvenirs, they're badges. Proof that you've stared down your battles, flipped them the bird, and come back tougher.

Think about your own hard-earned marks, what did they teach you? Because that's where the magic happens, tucked in the lessons between the stitches.

Rides can go both ways. I recall a midnight breakdown ride. My body had betrayed me again, and I couldn't make it home. I sat on the side of the road in tears, helmet off, head in my hands. Before I could call anyone, two bikes pulled up, sisters I'd only met once at a rally. They didn't ask what was wrong. They just parked, sat cross-legged on the asphalt, and kept me company until I could breathe again. Then one swung a leg over my bike and rode it home for me while the other followed with hazard lights flashing. They didn't leave until they saw me safe inside. That's sisterhood! Strangers until the moment you break, then family forever.

Being a biker woman means walking a different path. We wear patches that tell tales of loyalty, strength, and defiance. Every scar we carry is like a badge of honor, a reminder that we've survived challenges that others might shy away from. Whether it's dealing with the ups and downs of riding or standing strong against judgment, these experiences make us who we are.
No Bullshit Women.

So which scars can you flip from pain to pride? Maybe it's the one from a bad fall off your bike that taught you how to pick yourself up. Or perhaps it's the emotional scars from relationships that didn't work out but made you realize your worth. Each mark signifies courage and resilience, not weakness. Have you survived domestic violence, childhood abuse and found yourself stronger?

In our world, where society's cookie-cutter rules often crash headfirst into the biker code, owning your story is an act of defiance, and grace. Embrace your scars, loud and proud, and you're telling the world you own every bit of you. The raw, the rough, and the rebellious. Trust me, there's nothing more empowering than riding shotgun with your own story and laughing in the face of the fire that tried to burn you down.

The ride doesn't erase the pain. It transforms it.

What the world tried to bury, the road brings back to life.

And every time I ride, I rise.

Riding gave me resurrection. But resurrection isn't just for me; it's for the ones who come after. The daughters. The sisters. The ones who will carry the patch of fire into tomorrow.

So, here's your homework, no boring lectures, promise. Just really think about your questions this chapter.

Chapter 17 Legacy Reflection Questions

1. What's your version of wind therapy? Where do you go or what do you do when you need to breathe again and tell your demons to take a hike?

2. Have you ever felt closer to someone you've lost while cruising down the highway or sitting quietly in nature?

3. What did that fleeting moment teach you about life and loss?

"SISTERHOOD TEACHES YOU HOW TO SURVIVE THE MOMENT.

LEGACY TEACHES YOU HOW TO SURVIVE YOURSELF."

CHAPTER 18: LEGACY IN MOTION

"We ride for the versions of each other we're still becoming."

So here we are. You made it to the end of my story, which means you either really like me, or you're stuck in an elevator with no escape. Either way, thank you for sticking through the twists, turns, faceplants, and occasional "aha!" moments.

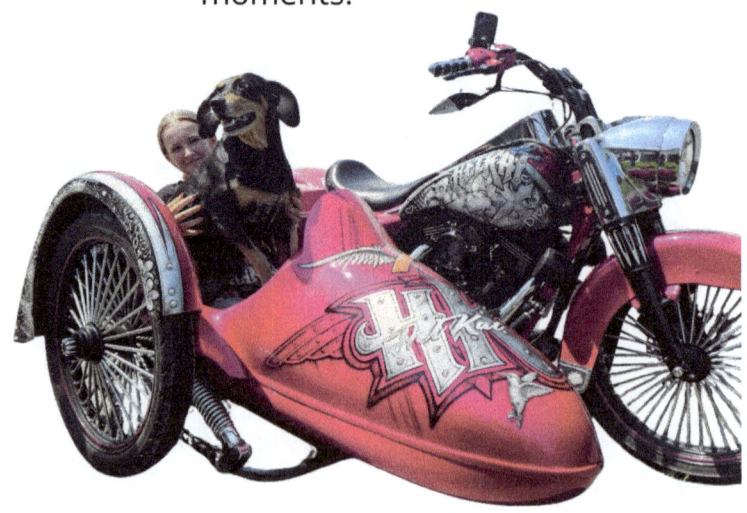

This isn't just my journey. It's a spotlight on the roads we all travel, often bumpy, sometimes hilarious, and always shared. This story isn't just mine. It's ours. I want you to share your story. I want you to grow from this book.

Legacy isn't about being stuck in some dusty rerun of the past. It's about grabbing the pen, flipping the script, and rewriting the whole damn story. You own story.

And personal growth? It's not a solo sport. No one "levels up" alone. We're all passengers on this crazy ride, clutching our stories like tickets, trying to make sense of the world and our place in it. What makes a story worth telling, or retelling, isn't the "me." It's the we. I got your six! Sisterhood!

Think about it. When you share what you've been through, you're not just narrating a chapter of your life, you're handing someone else a mirror, a roadmap, and maybe even a pair of binoculars for the horizon beyond their current view. You're translating your experiences into universal language, breaking cultural codes and rewiring old narratives with fresh hope.

This book wasn't written just to say, "Look what happened to me!", although, believe me, plenty happened. It's a rallying cry for all the riders, fighters, and believers tangled in the shared thread of human experience. We don't need to just endure; we need to blaze trails. And true translation? It's not just about swapping words. It's about **lighting fires**.

Yes, you still have a flame girl.

Fires Worth Lighting

True translation isn't about swapping words. After a betrayal split the club, I swore I'd never go back to a rally.

Too many ghosts, too much pain. But the women had other plans. They patched together a fundraiser under our own name with no men needed.

We sold t-shirts, raffled off baskets, and by the end of the night raised enough money to cover a sister's chemo. That night, I realized the truth. We weren't just supporting the sisterhood. We were the backbone of the damn culture.

So, what's next? This is your invitation, to lend your story, your voice, your truth. I pray you are stronger and empowered to rise above all triumphs.

That's why I started Biker Boss Kids, storytelling, books, and community programs rolling together like the ultimate crew. Breaking cycles? That's a hard solo ride. Building something stronger together? Now that's the real thrill.

Enter the Biker Boss Kids series. Where storytelling, books, and community programs team up like the ultimate biker crew to rewrite the narrative for the next generation. Because of breaking the cycle? That's a hell of a solo ride. Building something stronger together? Now that's the real thrill.

The Quiet Breaking

There's a moment in every biker woman's life when the ride gets quiet. Not because the engine died but because you did. Not literally. But emotionally. Spiritually. That silence is where betrayal, illness, and doubt all try to strip you bare.

This isn't about belonging to a club. It's about finding a rescue squad for your spirit. It's the women who show up when you're at your lowest, who understand the terrain because they've crashed and recovered on it, too. They don't just offer support, they share the wisdom earned through their own wrecks, guiding you back to the road with compassion and strength. In that silence, far from the roar of any V-Twin engine, something louder emerges; the sisterhood.

Sisterhood Ain't for Show

I've been burned by women who called me "sis" one day and cut me the next. I've walked into clubhouses invisible, dragged down by illness, left behind when I couldn't keep pace.
But the real sisterhood? She's the one who taps the brakes, so you can catch your breath without falling off. She looks you dead in the eye and says, *"Hell yes, that's the kind of woman I ride with, scratches, scars, sass, and all."*

Building the Next Legacy

I've seen women tear each other down when power clashed with insecurity. I've felt betrayal in circles that were supposed to feel safe. But I've also seen the toughest rise up, blazing their own trails, crafting their own tables, and inviting only those who bring respect.

So here's the deal;

- Own your damn name like you own your bike.
- Rock your patch without losing your voice.
- Strut with grit and class fierce enough to rattle chains.

Because sisterhood isn't glitter and group hugs. It's survival and fire.

Ol' lady Wisdom: Earned, Not Inherited

New around here? Hey, don't be shy. No, really, reach out. Because we've been around these roads, and trust me, we remember the jitters. Feeling like the rookie who can't keep pace, or worse, the invisible passenger stuck in the backseat. Most experienced ol' ladies will show you the ropes if you ask. We'll tell you what's expected, what's earned, and what to watch out for.

And we'll damn sure remind you that wearing a "Property Of" patch doesn't mean you disappear. It means you've stepped into something ancient, something sacred, something that has carried women through decades of pain, power, and purpose. You're not just claimed. You're claiming your place in a world built on honor. When you wear that patch with some serious swagger, it shows you've got loyalty not just to him, but to yourself, and every badass sister riding alongside you.

Let's get real, sisterhood isn't always glitter and group hugs. Sometimes the patch comes with pressure, competition, or side-eyes you can feel even behind your shades. There's a quiet war that can unfold when power meets insecurity, and sadly, some women forget the weight that comes with wearing their jacket.

This section is about calling that out. About making space for women who are ready to be real about their pain, ready to repair the sisterhood, and never again pretend everything's fine when it's not.

"Sisterhood ain't for show. It's earned, it's sacred, and it's stronger when we stop faking it."

The Soul of the Sisterhood

This isn't just about mastering the throttle or navigating curves. It's about ascending, united.

We build each other up with impromptu parking lot pep talks and late-night "call me, I'm losing it" calls. We show up at rallies, charity rides, and hold candlelight vigils for the ones who've ridden on ahead. We raise cash for breast cancer and hand-deliver food baskets to veterans, sometimes while munching fries post-ride, because, folks, it's all about balance.

When a sister loses her man, we show up with dignity and dirty jokes (because grief is better shared over laughter and leather). We ride together. We cry together. We rebuild together.

Our community is full of loud laughter, fierce love, and real conversations. We share survival stories, marriage lessons, club dynamics, motherhood chaos, and unfiltered truths. Because out here, we don't just ride for the lifestyle.
We ride for life.

Owning Your Name

If I could stash a gift in every woman's saddlebag, it'd be this, **Own your damn name like you own your bike.** You can be someone's ol' lady and still be your own force. You can wear a patch without losing your voice. You can ride with scars, broken bones, or a body that feels like it betrayed you and still blaze the road with more power than anyone who doubted you.

We celebrate individuality here.
We lift women up, whether they ride their own or ride passenger.
We offer guidance, not gossip.
Wisdom, not warnings.
Because we want you to thrive. To stand tall in your boots, damn it. To know your worth before anyone else tries slapping a bargain-bin price tag on it. To know your worth before someone else defines it for you.

The Biker Sisterhood & The Ride-or-Dies

Alright, let's break this down. When we talk about "ride-or-dies," we're diving into something real and deep. These are the women who stand by you when life gets messy, when the road gets bumpy, and everything feels off-kilter. But here's the kicker. Before you can figure out who your ride-or-dies are, you've got to ask yourself if you're a ride-or-die for yourself.

It means surrounding yourself with those who respect your strength and loyalty, the kind of bonds that don't snap under pressure. Think of it like building your own biker sisterhood; it doesn't just happen overnight. You've got to invest time and heart in these relationships, just like you would in customizing your bike or mastering a challenging curve on the open road.

So, let's get honest. Who's in your corner? Are they lifting you up, reminding you of your fierce HelKat spirit? Or do they pull you down with their doubts and negativity? Maybe it's time to weed out the ones who don't honor the code of loyalty and respect.

And how about you?
I've buried brothers. I've fought illness. I've lost people I thought would never leave. And yet here I am. Still loud. Still standing. Still riding.

This is the roar I leave you with,
Don't wait for permission. Don't shrink for comfort. Don't let anyone else write your story.

Take the throttle. Ride your truth. Start something new.
And that's why we're here, behind the patch. Not just to tell my story, but to roar a legacy loud enough that no one forgets the women who carried it.

Chapter 18 Legacy Reflection Questions

1. What legacy do you want to leave behind and is it loud enough yet?

2. Who in your circle deserves to carry the fire with you, and who do you need to release?

3. If you could build one thing; book, business, ride, or ritual that reflects your soul, what would it be?

4. What does "starting something new" look like in your life right now?

5. What roar will you leave behind so no one forgets you were here?

FINAL CHAPTER: NEVER JUST A PASSENGER

"This story won't end with me. It begins with the next woman who dares."

You made it to the end of this ride. If you've stuck with me through chrome, chaos, cancer, club codes, and callouts, then I know you're not just a Sunday reader. You're someone who wants to understand real stories.

They're the wild and wonderful ones, the women with burn scars and beauty marks. These are the daring souls who ride out the storms, spilling secrets that time forgot.

Roaring down the open highway, they carry values as big as their hearts, rooted in honor and devotion. It's all about living life their way. Among ol' ladies, these women thrive, crafting connections that warm the soul and defy the odds.
You see, biker life isn't about faking toughness.

Life can hit like a freight train, and sometimes it feels like the universe is out to get you. Yet, there are phenomenal women facing their battles head-on while raising their kids. There are men who weep at funerals, then quietly get their hands greasy rebuilding engines. These tales showcase the power of found family and rock-solid loyalty.

In a world quick to judge, these rebels live by their own compass, carving out a code of honor that steers them through life's hurdles. It's about those heartwarming moments that shine through the shadows and the confessions we tuck away.

So when life throws a curveball or obstacles block the road, remember the art of thriving against the odds. Embrace your path and stand tall in adversity, because everyone has a story worth telling.

Me?

I've lived many lives. I've been the supportive partner, a fearless rider, and a survivor through tough times. Behind the scenes, I've kept everything running smoothly while the loud engines roar in front of me. I've worn lipstick with my leather jacket, faced loss by burying friends, and found strength in writing books. People have often underestimated me, misjudged my health, or simply ignored what I could do, but they've never managed to erase my story.

As a woman in this world, I've learned about loyalty and honor among those who share the same passion for motorcycles.

The challenges I've faced haven't stopped me. With every confession and shocking twist along the way, I've stayed devoted to my values and the rules that guide us. My journey is heartwarming, full of lessons learned and new roads taken.

This book isn't a tell-all. It's a reclaiming.

It's me saying; ***"I see the good. I survived the bad. And I'm here to tell the damn truth."***

Motorcycle clubs are complex AF.

The ones I grew up around were both protectors and predators, builders and bruisers. And some? Just people trying to find their way like the rest of us. So don't flatten these lives into soundbites. Don't call a community a "gang" just because you don't understand it.

And for the love of all things holy, don't tell a woman like me to sit on the back seat unless I damn well want to.

Because here's the truth, I was never meant to ride behind anyone.

I was born to ride beside the best of them.

Final Chapter Legacy Reflection Questions

1. What parts of your story deserve to be told, even if no one claps?

2. What spaces are you done apologizing for taking up?

3. If you had to leave one mark on this world, what would your "patch" say?

NOW IT'S YOUR TURN

To write a story that makes others feel like they're not alone, you need to dig deep into the heart of what it means to be a woman in a world filled with rules and expectations. This isn't just about leather jackets and roaring engines; it's about the battles we fight every day, the silent struggles and loud victories.

So what's your road? Where do you need to roar louder? Where do you need to set fire to the silence? Don't just read this book and put it down like another chapter closed. Pick up the throttle of your own life. Ride it raw. Ride it loud. Ride it honest.

Because survival is one thing. Legacy is another. And your legacy starts the moment you decide to stop shrinking.
Start by reflecting on your own journey. What challenges did you face when stepping into this wild biker life? Share those moments! Readers connect through honesty, so don't shy away from your confessions, those times when you thought you were lost but found your way instead.

Write about the incredible women who've come before you. Talk about the values that drive these fierce souls: loyalty, courage, and passion. Let them know they are part of something bigger, a legacy woven together with strength and spirit.

But don't just stick to the good stuff. Life is messy and complicated. Address the strange and unbelievable moments too, the times when it all seemed too much. Those experiences create bonds between readers because everyone has faced odds.

THE FINAL RIDE

Engines cool. Roads fade. But the ride never really ends. This is where the book ends, but not where the ride does.
Picture it: the road stretched out ahead, sun dropping low, chrome catching fire in the light. The scars are still there, but so is the roar in your chest. The wind doesn't erase the pain, it teaches you how to carry it.

We ride for the versions of each other we're still becoming. And if you remember nothing else from my story, remember this:

You belong here. Your scars are proof you survived. Your voice is the throttle. And the legacy you're building?

It's already rumbling down the road.

So start it. Ride it. Live it. Loud. Every ride is a prayer. Every mile is proof.

And this one?

This one's yours.

♥ LEGACY REFLECTION

Not This. Not on My Watch.

There's a part of my story I didn't want to tell. Not because I'm ashamed, but because I knew once it hit the page, I could never pretend it didn't shape me.

I've lived through things that tried to bury me. Cancer, lupus, MS, divorce, betrayal, biker politics, broken systems, broken bones, and broken hearts. And I kept going. Not just because I'm strong, but because I had no damn choice.

Some days, I wasn't a warrior, I was a woman whispering to herself in the mirror:

"Get through this. Just one more day. Don't let them win."
And now? I speak from the other side of the storm. Not fully healed. Not perfectly wise. But wide awake and wide open.

So let me say this clearly, for the ones still walking your road:

You don't have to shrink to survive.
You don't have to be quiet to be respected.
You don't have to be perfect, to be powerful.

Pain: Do you ever feel like you're constantly putting everyone else first, while your own needs get lost in the shuffle? You flip the script for everyone else, juggling kids, keeping the house spotless, and making sure the fundraisers run smoothly, yet, deep down, you're unraveling.

Agitate: Imagine the weight of those unreciprocated sacrifices crushing your spirit, day after day.

It's frustrating to say yes when your gut is screaming "No."

You find yourself doing it out of loyalty to people who wouldn't even stop to help you in your toughest times. In the motorcycle world, where rules and honor are everything, it's shocking how easily some forget what really matters. We're told to stand by our brothers and sisters no matter what, but that doesn't mean we should ignore our own needs or feelings.

And if you take anything from this book, let it be this:

- You don't owe anyone your pain in a pretty package.
- You get to outgrow who they thought you were.
- You are allowed to be soft and steel at the same time.

And you?

You're not alone.

With pride,
HelKat

These aren't chapter-specific. They're life-specific.
Sit with them. Don't rush.

1. What roar will you leave behind so no one forgets you were here?

2. Who in your life has proven true loyalty and who needs to be cut loose?

3. What fire inside you refuses to die, no matter what storms hit?

4. If you could write one truth on the sky for the next generation, what would it say?

5. What does "legacy" mean to you, not someday, but right now?

♥ DEAR YOUNGER ME,

Girl, I see you. You won't always feel this lost. Sitting in that cold hospital room at 3 a.m., pretending not to cry.
Standing outside that bar fight, clutching rage in one hand and fear in the other.
Wondering if you'll ever be enough. Here's the truth, you were always enough. You just didn't know it yet.
The pain? It shaped you. The scars? They became your ink.
The storms? They made you loud.
So don't you dare give up. Don't you dare let them write you small.
Because one day, you'll be me. You'll be HelKat.
And you'll roar so loud the whole damn world will hear.
You'll love people who don't deserve you and fight battles no one claps for, but you will survive every one of them.
And you'll become someone who fights not just for herself, but for every other girl who didn't know she had a voice.
Stop shrinking to fit into rooms that weren't built for your power.
Start believing that your pain isn't the end of your story, it's the fire that will forge it.
You'll ride one day, on steel, on strength, on your own terms.
I'm proud of you. Even when you couldn't see a future, you kept going.
Keep going,
Me

♥ THE PATCH ISN'T JUST HIS
IT'S OURS TOO.

For too long, women in biker culture have been written as passengers, property, background noise to a story we've been carrying just as hard as any man.
But the truth is this: the patch isn't just his. It's ours too.
We've earned it in silence, in sacrifice, in fire no one else wanted to touch. We've raised kids in clubhouses, buried brothers, held secrets, healed wounds, and carried legacies without credit.
And now? We're not asking. We're claiming.
We are the women who ride alongside, lead from the front, and hold the line when others fold. We are not property. We are presence.
We claim our stories. Our scars.
Our seats at the table.
We speak with fire. We love with grit.
We rise with purpose.
We protect our own,
but we never forget to protect ourselves.
We are not here to be quiet.
We are here to be legendary.
This is our manifesto.
This is our patch.

♥WHAT YOU MIGHT HAVE MISSED

Behind the stories, scars, and sisterhood is a blueprint for how to rise without apology.
You didn't just read about riding,
you read about reclaiming.
About daring to tell the truth even when the world would rather you smile pretty and stay quiet.
You read about a woman who learned to trust herself after the world made her doubt everything.
You may have thought this book was about motorcycles and patches, but it's really about power.
And the choice to stop handing it away.
If you missed that, go back.
Start again.
This time, read it as if your life depends on it,
because maybe your freedom does.

- Brotherhood is holy. Betrayal is hell.
- Every scar is a story. Every story deserves a roar.
- The road doesn't erase pain. It transforms it.
- Legacy isn't whispered. It's shouted.
- The patch isn't just his. It's ours too.

♥FINAL AFFIRMATION PAGE

· I am storm-born.
· I am scarred.
· I am still here.
· I am not a passenger.
· I ride.

♥ I am the voice I needed when I was silent.
♥ I ride for the woman I've become, not the ones who left.
♥ I don't owe anyone pretty or polite. I owe myself peace.
♥ My scars are not shameful. They are survival stories.
♥ I am not for everyone. I am for the brave.
♥ I rise for my daughters and the ones who never got the chance.
♥ I am both: a rebel and a reflection.
♥ I won't shrink to be loved, I will roar to be heard.

"HELKAT'S TRANSLATOR BOOTH"

Because let's be real, Google Translate doesn't speak "biker."

Purpose:
This glossary is your unofficial tour guide through the twisty alleys of biker slang and feminist buzzwords.

Think of it as your trusty pit stop where jargon gets defanged and cultural references are demystified, all served with a side of sass and a wink. It's inexpensive, quick, and guaranteed to induce chuckles (or at least a well-timed smirk). More importantly, it reaffirms your role as the cool, bilingual bridge between the road warriors and the change-makers.

- **Patch**: A badge of belonging. Earned, never handed.
- **Cut**: The vest — sacred garment of the MC world.
- **Ol' lady**: Partner to a patched member. Title can mean respect, pressure, or both. Signify Love, Commitment.
- **Prospect**: A hopeful. A rookie. A soul getting tested by fire.
- **Brotherhood/Sisterhood**: Family, sometimes stronger than blood. Sometimes not.
- **Ride-or-die**: Exactly what it sounds like. No half-measures.

1. **Babes on Bikes**
Literal Meaning: Women who ride motorcycles.
Translator Notes: Not just decorative seat warmers or fuel gauges. These ladies mean business and torque. Bonus points if they can fix a flat tire faster than you can say "gas station espresso." Not your average "passenger with a helmet". These ladies don't just ride pillion, they dominate the asphalt with style and grit. Whether tearing up highways or joining rides for social justice, they are a crucial part of biker culture and feminist empowerment. Think of them as queens of torque and tenacity with a side of "don't mess with me."

2. **The Sisterhood**
Literal Meaning: A group of women bonded by feminism or female biker camaraderie.
Translator Notes: Think less "Mean Girls," more "Warriors in Leather Jackets." They're united by solidarity, shared battles, and occasionally shared cupcakes after a long ride or a hard-fought protest.

3. **Chrome and Courage**
Literal Meaning: The shiny, chrome parts of a bike and the bravery needed to ride.
Translator Notes: Because only a fearless soul can love the smell of gasoline in the morning and the roar of an engine that loud before coffee. Wear both pride badges with grit and grin.

4. **Patriarchy Pit Stop**
Literal Meaning: Moments or situations where patriarchal norms slow feminist progress.
Translator Notes: Don't get comfortable here. Refuel on patience, challenge the status quo, and maybe pop a sarcastic one-liner or two before getting back on the road. That awkward moment when society tries to slow you down. Like a literal rest area sign flashing "Welcome to Mansplainville," it's a place of frustration, but also reflection. Use this time to regroup, strategize, and roar back onto the highway of equality.

5. **Leather and Liberation**
Literal Meaning: The biker's second skin and a metaphor for feminist freedom.
Translator Notes: It's tough, flexible, and looks badass, just like the women who wear it and the ideals they ride for.

6. **Revving the Revolution**
Literal Meaning: Combining the loud, rebellious spirit of biking with activist energy.
Translator Notes: Imagine a motorcycle engine's growl waking people up to gender equality. Loud? Yes. Effective? Absolutely.

7. **Gearhead Gurus**
Literal Meaning: Those who know everything about motorcycle mechanics.
Translator Notes: They'll fix your bike and school you on feminist theory if you ask nicely. Or if you come bearing coffee.

8. **Biker Babble**
Literal Meaning: The unique set of slang, acronyms, and inside jokes shared by bikers.
Translator Notes: Words like "chunking," "throttle," and "bobber" aren't made-up spells. Use the HelKat's Booth to decode before you nod wisely.

9. **Feminist Fireroad**
Literal Meaning: The path less traveled, full of obstacles and potential surprises.
Translator Notes: Taking this route means embracing uncertain roads with grit and laughter, because both feminism and off-roading can get bumpy.

10. **The Road Warrior's Manifesto**
Literal Meaning: The guiding principles of feminist bikers.
Translator Notes: Equal rights, open road, open minds. Expect a blend of leather, logic, and an unapologetic sense of justice.

11. **Biker Lingo Basics**
 - Hangin' Loose: Not just a casual attitude, it's the art of rolling with the road and the chaos.
 - Burnout: More than a work hazard; it's a smokey tire dance that's biker poetry.
 - Patch Holder: The VIP member, whose vest is basically their résumé.

12. **Feminist Terminology 101**
 - Smashing the Patriarchy: No actual smashing required, though a sledgehammer might be tempting. It's about dismantling systemic oppression.
 - Gaslighting: When someone rewires your reality, so you're left wondering if your coffee was ever hot. Spoiler: It was.
 - Intersectionality: Like a kaleidoscope of identity, it's complicated but worth the view.

13. **Cultural Touchstones Decoded**
 - Leather vs. Lace: Not just fashion choices, but revolutionary armor and elegant defiance.
 - The Road as Sister: Why bikers say, "ride hard, ride free", and why feminists liken it to their fight for autonomy.

14. **Common Misconceptions, Busted**
 - "Biker culture is all tattoos and tough-guy posturing." Nope, that's just Act One. Act Two involves deep community and unexpected tenderness.
 - "Feminism means man-hating." Nope again. More like equality with a side of kick-ass confidence.

15. **Quirky Expressions for the Win**
 - Grip it and Rip It: Not advice for pottery class, but how to take life's handlebars with gusto.
 - Riding Sisterhood: It's not a bike route, it's a movement.

16. **HelKat's Personal Anecdotes**
 - Short, punchy tales that illustrate terms in action, because jargon makes so much more sense when there's a wild story behind it.

DEDICATED TO THE WOMEN WHO RIDE

For my three girls

You are the fire that kept me alive when the road tried to break me.
This book is my roar, but it's also your inheritance.
May you ride louder, freer, and braver than I ever did.
To the ones who kept riding after heartbreak, after diagnosis, after betrayal.
To the daughters becoming legends.
To the ol' ladies who paved the way.
To the rebels, survivors, and storm-bringers.
You are not just part of the patchwork,
You are the thread that holds it together.
Ride on,
HelKat ♥

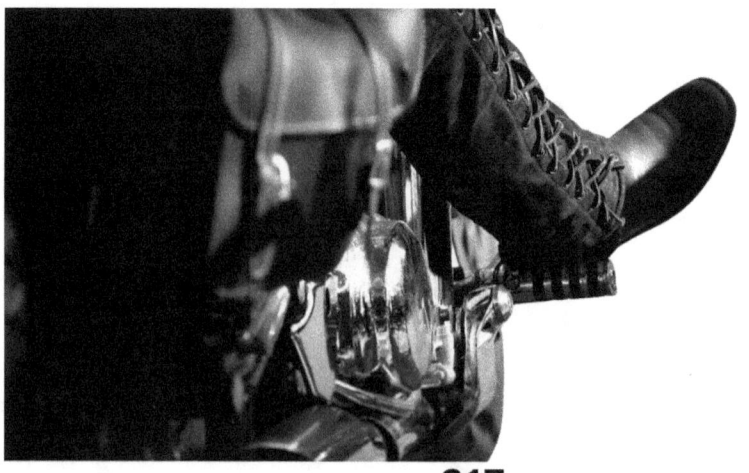

Through my books, fearless coaching, and vibrant presence in the biker community, let's empower women to reclaim their strength, voice their truths, and live life on their own terms.
Here's a toolbox brimming with resilience, a heart ablaze with passion, and a powerful message: You don't need to be flawless to be formidable.

🖤 Still standing. Still roaring. Still riding.
[www.helkatreflections.com] (http://www.helkatreflections.com)
✉ bikerbosscoaching@gmail.com
📍 York County, PA

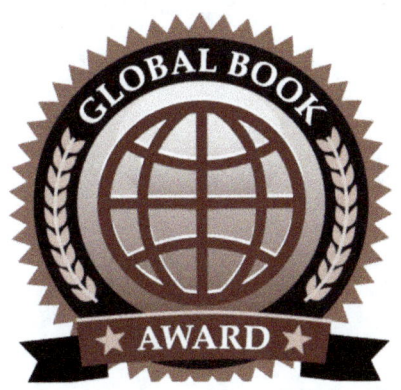

ACKNOWLEDGMENTS

To every woman who ever swallowed her voice,
This book is for you.

To my daughters, who teach me how to be softer without breaking, and to speak love even in war,
You are my legacy.

To the biker sisterhood, especially the ones who don't flinch at hard truths or hard roads,
Thank you for holding space for my evolution, even when I had to ride alone for a while.
To the ones who doubted me,
You gave me fuel.
To the ones who lifted me,
You gave me wings.

And to my Creator, who saw the warrior in the woman long before I picked up a pen,
Thank you for this mission. I'm still riding it.

Some of the emotional processing behind this book also found its way into music written during the same period.

With love, rage, and gratitude,
HelKat

―――― HELKAT LEGACY CO. ――――

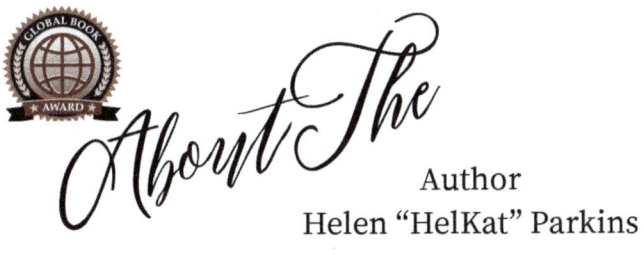
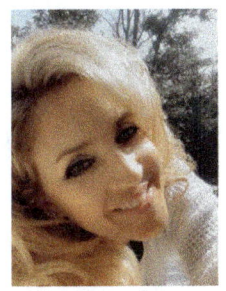

About The Author
Helen "HelKat" Parkins

I am a proud biker, mother, survivor, and unapologetic force of nature. Raised in the wind and hardened by life's fires, I have lived loudly with a rebel heart and a backbone built on faith and sisterhood.

By day, I'm a program analyst, but deep down, I'm the boss of my own bike world. I ride through life with my chrome-coated story, a tale that's tough, real, and packed with stories that most never endure in a lifetime.

Hello friends, I've faced cancer head-on and live every day with multiple sclerosis and lupus, yet here I am, still riding harder than most.

Life has thrown me some serious challenges, and trust me, there have been moments that would leave anyone shaken. But instead of letting those struggles define me, I've learned to embrace them. Each scar tells a story, and each bump in the road has only made me stronger.

In this club life, we have our rules and codes, honor among bikers, loyalty as strong as leather, but what truly matters is how we treat each other. As women in this world, we face unique battles, often feeling forgotten or overshadowed. It's time we change that narrative.

I'm all about empowerment, especially for women navigating their own twists and turns. Whether it's dealing with illness, trauma, or just trying to find your place in a male-dominated space, know that you're not alone. We can thrive together, supporting one another while living loudly and not for pity. I am here to speak the truth.

www.ingramcontent.com/pod-product-compliance
Lightning Source LLC
LaVergne TN
LVHW081455060526
838201LV00051BA/1806